# Common and Uncommon Scents

# COMMON AND UNCOMMON SCENTS
## A SOCIAL HISTORY OF PERFUME

SUSAN STEWART

AMBERLEY

'The history of perfume is in some manner the
history of civilisation.'

Eugene Rimmel,
*The Book of Perfume* (1865)

First published 2022

Amberley Publishing
The Hill, Stroud
Gloucestershire, GL5 4EP

www.amberley-books.com

Copyright © Susan Stewart, 2022

The right of Susan Stewart to be identified as
the Author of this work has been asserted in
accordance with the Copyright, Designs and
Patents Act 1988.

ISBN 978 1 4456 9318 7 (hardback)
ISBN 978 1 4456 9319 4 (ebook)

British Library Cataloguing in Publication Data.
A catalogue record for this book is available
from the British Library.

1 2 3 4 5 6 7 8 9 10

Typesetting by SJmagic DESIGN SERVICES, India.
Printed in the UK.

# CONTENTS

I

# THE ESSENCE OF PERFUME

Smell is a potent wizard that transports you across thousands of
miles and all the years you have lived.

Helen Keller (1880–1968)

Of our five senses, smell is the most basic, something that has
been integral to our existence from our very beginnings.
Prehistoric man used his sense of smell to detect danger and to
find food. As a result smell is sometimes dismissed, even shunned,
as too base, too animal to warrant our attention. This is a view
expressed by philosophers from Plato to Kant. Modern scholars
think differently, though, looking instead at the senses (arguably
smell in particular) as a route to a better understanding of the
past. We know how powerful smell can be; it is very closely linked
to our feelings, our emotions and our memory. This is a scientific
fact that can be anatomically explained. Catching even a whiff
of a certain fragrance can instantly remind us of a particular
childhood memory, a special person or place. Today, sensory
history is a valued and rewarding area of historical research.

## What Is a Perfume?
This book focuses on smell as it pertains to a largely pleasant
scent – a perfume, or fragrance if you like. It is important,

however, to remember that what smells good is always subjective. It is also true to say that the general definition of a pleasant smell has not remained static over time. What is meant by the very words 'scent' and 'perfume' has changed too. So, what *do* we mean by a scent or a perfume? The *Oxford English Dictionary* gives us the following definition of the word scent: 'A distinctive smell, especially one that is pleasant ... a pleasant-smelling liquid worn on the skin; perfume.' The definition of the word perfume from the same source is as follows: 'The fragrance or odour emitted by any (usually pleasant-smelling) substance or thing ... a fragrant liquid, usually consisting of aromatic ingredients (natural or synthetic) in a base of alcohol, used to impart a pleasant smell to the body, clothes, etc.' It is acknowledged that the word 'perfume' originally referred to a substance that emitted a pleasant smell when burned. This is particularly relevant as the word perfume itself does not make an appearance until 1546 and is derived from the Latin *per fumum*, which, taken literally, means 'through smoke' – in other words, incense.

For us the word perfume probably conjures up an image of a liquid in a bottle. Historically speaking, nothing could be further from the truth. Scent, or fragrance, or perfume, has not always been a liquid. Before the Middle Ages perfume was more commonly a solid, based on fats or oils impregnated with the scent of plant or perhaps animal matter. It is only from around the seventeenth century onwards that we find liquid perfumes beginning to take centre stage. By then, scent was more often made with an alcohol base and bears a much closer resemblance to the bottles of perfume we can buy today. Historically, however, the nature of scent, its use and the ideas associated with it were much broader in scope than a modern dictionary definition will allow. There is much more to be understood about the actual function of a fragrance, its composition, its meaning and its associations over the centuries.

## *The Purpose of Scent*

In the twenty-first century, the personal use of scent to make oneself attractive to others could be said to be the main function of fragrance. Perfume did make a fashion statement in the past, and could be used to bolster one's appeal, but it could also reflect a person's wealth and status, allowing the onlooker to distinguish an important person from one of low social standing, to identify an individual as belonging to a particular social group. In ancient societies perfume might even have been a means of distinguishing the divine from the human. Although in some places and at some times it was gender specific, for most of history it has been employed by both sexes. Personal preference played, and still plays, a key role in the appreciation of a particular scent and there were also passing fads and fashions.

Although the people of the past were accustomed to the use of fragrance as a means of adornment, it had many other uses too, only some of which are still relevant today. For example, it was useful for freshening the air, covering up personal body odour and counteracting unpleasant communal smells such as the stench of animal sacrifices at religious ceremonies or the reek of decay, disease and death during epidemics.

More specifically, in the ancient world as well as in the medieval and the early modern, one of the primary uses of perfume was as a medicine. Scent was understood to improve one's wellbeing mentally as well as physically, and before modern medical knowledge came into being it was believed to prevent disease. Nowadays we know that the fragrant properties of some herbs, flowers and spices may indeed have some medicinal benefit, hence their return in the form of alternative medicines and aromatherapy treatments. Suffice to say, the people of the past, though driven by necessity to rely on properties of plants (including their scent) as medicine, were not wholly wrong and can certainly be said to have done their best with what they had.

In addition to its function in masking bad smells, adding to personal attractiveness and curing illness, scent also played an important part in religious ritual. The burning of incense was a feature of religious ceremonies, festivals and events and therefore has close links not only with the divine but also with the idea of success and celebration both communal and personal, whether heralding the return of triumphant warriors or celebrating a family wedding. In pre-Christian times, people might be buried with scent bottles for use in the afterlife or simply as an indication of their social status. At the funeral itself, scent reverted to its basic function of concealing the offensive odour of death.

In short, religion, gender, health and healing, luxury and status, attraction, desire, love, emotion, memory and fashion, among other concepts, are closely associated with the use of scent on the body, on clothing and in interior and exterior spaces.

## Making a Perfume: The Basics

> [There are] two ingredients, the juice and the solid part, the former which usually consists of various sorts of oil and the latter of scented substances ... a sprinkle of salt serves to preserve the properties of the oil ... resin or gum are added to retain the scent in the solid part as it evaporates and disappears very quickly if these are not added.
>
> Pliny the Elder, *Historia Naturalis*

Perfumery is both an art and a science: a matter of chemistry and of aesthetics. A basic perfume is made from organic materials sourced from plants, animals or, from the middle of the nineteenth century, synthetic compounds that replicate them. Up until around 1340, when the first perfume using alcohol is thought to have been produced, the basic ingredients were oil or fat, an aromatic, a solvent or thinning agent (in which to suspend the scent) and a fixative to help the odour persist. Colour might also be added to make the finished product more appealing.

In the ancient world perfumes were based on fat, usually olive oil or balanos oil from the Egyptian plum tree, or maybe *omphacium*, an oil made from unripe grapes. Aromatics, such as sweet-smelling plants or fragrant woods, could be mixed with fat (a process known as enfleurage) or steeped in heated oil (a method known as maceration). Either way, the oil would take on the scent of the flowers or aromatics. The juices, or essential oil, of a particular fragrant plant might also be obtained by expression; that is, simply squeezing out the juice or oil such as one might do with citrus fruits. Finally, resin might be used as a fixative and colour could be added with natural dye such as madder or alkanet. These concoctions were thicker than modern perfumes, and greasy. If the mixture was too thick then a thinning agent such as wine or water might be added.

Today, perfume is manufactured using distillation in alcohol, a process perfected in the Middle Ages and which could be said to have revolutionised early perfume production. Where the ingredients were organic (flowers, leaves and the like) they would be put into a still and boiled with water to give off steam. Along with the steam, the essential oils of the plant would rise to the top of the still. As these cooled they turned to a liquid that could be siphoned off. The process allowed scent to be produced on a much larger scale than had been the case in previous centuries.

Modern perfumes consist of alcohol, essential oils (or their synthetic equivalents), fixatives, colouring and preservatives. Solvent extraction was developed in the early nineteenth century and involves the removal of essential oils from fragile flowers that cannot withstand distillation in a complicated and expensive process using wax to mop up the oils and then separating the two again. Chemists, meanwhile, developed synthetic substitutes for many natural perfumes. Additional modern techniques for creating a scent include headspace technology, which was developed in the 1980s and by which the chemical make-up of a live plant is analysed and replicated artificially. Today, a true perfume must contain at least 15 per cent essential oil diluted with alcohol. Colognes and toilet waters are weaker and must contain between 3 and 10 per cent.

## The Scent Trail

Historically, the source of many favoured plants for use in scents could be found in the civilisations of the Middle East. I will begin with descriptions of these early civilisations and their perfumes, turning then to the classical worlds of Greece and Rome that nurtured the practical use of scent and an appreciation of fragrance. From there I will follow the passage of perfume into western Europe through medieval Arabic medicine, religious observance and the social customs of Late Antiquity. These scents passed through trade, adoption of customs and the influence of eminent individuals into Europe, where first Italy and Spain, then France, and latterly Britain and America became centres of sought-after scents. The subject is vast, and so this volume must restrict itself; the use of scent in the specific cultures of India and China must await another book.

The nature of scent over the centuries developed in accord with changing times: the invention of processes, the availability of goods, the growth of cities and indeed fashion, fancy, personal preference and personal influence. Experiments in mixing scents together and the advancement of technology, the availability of new products and even the increased availability of established ingredients which allowed for cheaper goods to be produced in larger quantities all had an impact on how fragrance might be used. This book is not about how to make perfume (beyond the basics), nor is it simply a list of famous perfumes and their ingredients. Instead, the aim is to put scent in its true historical context, to explain how we can further understand societies of the past and indeed shed light on our own; to place scent in a social, economic, religious and even political context in order to stress the importance of fragrance as a way to interpret and hopefully better understand the past.

# 2

# THE ANCIENT WORLD
## Perfume, Priests and Palaces

'Take fragrant spices – gum resin, onycha and galbanum – and pure
frankincense, all in equal amounts.'

Exodus 30:34

Prior to any extant writing on the topic, archaeologists have
found material proof that aromatic oils were known and used
by early peoples. Evidence from prehistoric remains excavated
on the island of Cyprus suggests that birthing practices involved
scent: it has been proposed that aromatics were used to purify
the mother and her new baby. The size and shape of vessels
found at Neolithic sites in south-eastern Europe indicate
that these contained plant material including cedarwood,
juniper and cypress oil, possibly for use as incense. Modern
techniques such as gas spectrometry – a means of examining
the contents of containers without damaging the vessels
themselves – have revealed the presence of camphor and pine
resin, too. The earliest vessels thought to have contained
scent were excavated at various sites in Syria and are believed
to date from around 7000 BC. More evidence of the use of
aromatics was uncovered in a rock shelter in South Africa,
where archaeologists discovered a prehistoric mattress made of
layers of grasses, herbs and other plant material. The aromatic

leaves of the laurel tree which formed part of this grass mattress would have helped to prevent infestations of fleas. So, though the record is inevitably scant (we are, after all, talking about organic materials that break down easily and decay quickly), prehistoric peoples were certainly aware of fragrant plants that could be useful in their daily lives.

## The Bronze Age

The period of time referred to by historians as the Bronze Age begins around 3000 BC and lasts until approximately 1200 BC in the Near East, though it ends somewhat later in the West, around 700 BC. In the latter region it is subdivided into the Early (1800 BC–1600 BC), Middle (1600 BC–1200 BC) and Late (1300 BC–700 BC) Bronze Ages. Across these centuries a number of sophisticated civilisations came and went. Some overlapped in a temporal sense, and while they were geographically distant they were far from being mutually exclusive, engaging in trade both directly and indirectly.

First among these were the peoples living around the confluence of the rivers Tigris and Euphrates, the area that covers southern Iraq and Kuwait today. From the classical period at least, this area was known as Mesopotamia, literally (in Ancient Greek) 'the land between two rivers'. Mesopotamia comprised a number of city states. We refer to the best known of the peoples that lived there as the Sumerians. Their society prospered from around 4500 BC until about 1900 BC and was superseded by that of the Amorites, founders of the ancient city of Mari (on the west bank of the Euphrates) and the first dynasty of the Babylonian Empire.

Meanwhile, the Minoans, another Bronze Age civilisation, prospered on the island of Crete from around 3000 BC to 1100 BC, and on mainland Greece the Mycenaeans lived a refined lifestyle from around 1600 to 1200 BC. The Phoenicians, who had settled on a narrow coastal strip between the Mount Lebanon range and the Mediterranean Sea, were another developing nation thriving from around 1550 BC to 300 BC. They were industrious traders and undoubtedly helped to distribute luxury products including scent from east to west and vice versa. Penultimately, we have the Ancient Egyptians whose history we divide chronologically into the Old (2700 BC–2200 BC), Middle (2050 BC–1800 BC), and New (about 1550 BC–1100 BC) Kingdoms. Finally, around 550 BC, tagging on to the very end of the Bronze Age, the Persians established a great empire in what is now Iran. For all these societies, scent served an important role in both public and private life.

## The First Writing

With the dawning of the Bronze Age, we enter a period which has left us a written record. Although inevitably it is fragmentary, this material is extremely valuable. It covers a range of different genres, including administrative texts, financial accounts, medical manuals and religious documents. In all of these contexts, scent crops up on a regular basis and we are given a sense not only of its typical composition but also of its value, its importance and its many uses.

The Sumerians developed a writing system consisting of angular, wedge-shaped lines which we call cuneiform. They wrote on clay tablets which they then hardened in the sun. The tablets at any given site are generally a record from one particular year because the Sumerians softened and reused the clay annually. There are thousands of these tablets, providing us with a record of industrial activity and financial transactions where aromatics feature significantly as items that were bought and sold on a regular basis.

The Minoans and Mycenaeans wrote in versions of early Greek known to us as Linear A and Linear B. Linear A is still a mystery but the tablets written in Linear B were deciphered, to much acclaim, by the British architect, classicist and philologist Michael Ventris in the 1950s. Scent features here, too, particularly in palace accounts and records of religious offerings. The Ancient

Egyptians are of course famous for their hieroglyphs, and in their writing perfumes feature prominently as offerings to the gods, treatments for disease and as tools for protection against evil spirits, as well as the more mundane purposes of keeping oneself clean and making oneself beautiful.

## Scent in Art and Archaeology

While we have certainly benefited from being able to understand, in large part, the writing of these early civilisations, our evidence for the use of scent in the Bronze Age is not only to be found in the written record. Works of art and archaeological remains offer many clues to the part scent played in everyday life. Minoan and Ancient Egyptian wall paintings depict the harvesting of aromatic plants as well as illustrating the role of scent in ancient ceremony through incense burners and other related objects.

The jars, bottles and other vessels used to transport, store and dispense these perfumes are frequent finds at archaeological sites. Some of these vessels are very elaborate, intended not only for practical use but as a symbol of their owners' wealth and power. Others are simpler, perhaps for more everyday use or maybe the possessions of a less wealthy household. Containers are regularly found in both domestic and funerary contexts, in the case of the latter being either buried with the body or discarded among the detritus after use at the funeral ceremony itself.

Archaeologists have also excavated large numbers of vessels alongside other perfume-making equipment, such as vats and presses, at sites where perfume appears to have been produced on a large scale not only for use by those living in the immediate environs but sufficient for export and trade as well. If enough residue can be extracted it is sometimes possible to analyse the contents of the vessels to find out more about what these ancient perfumes were made of and potentially to even recreate them. We should bear in mind, however, that no matter how accurate we can be in replicating an ancient perfume the popular preferences of the past are not necessarily the same as our own. We must also consider how these fragrances would have mixed with the other, often strong smells that would have filled the air in the home and outside it. Replicating an ancient scent and interpreting the result is far from being an exact science.

## Incense: The First Perfume

Scent was first deployed in the form of incense, whereby an aromatic gum resin or wood bark, such as frankincense, myrrh or cedarwood, was burnt to give off a pleasant smell. The word incense refers both to the material itself and to the scent released when this is set alight, coming from the Latin *incendere*, meaning 'to set on fire'.

For the peoples of the ancient world the aromatic smell produced was imbued with considerable spiritual significance. The religions followed by the Sumerians, Minoans, Mycenaeans, and Ancient Egyptians were all pantheistic; that is to say, these peoples worshipped many different gods who had specific responsibilities for various aspects of everyday life. Scent played an integral part in religious ceremonies honouring these gods. In fact, it may have been a feature of religious observance at the very erection of a sacred building. Aromatics were often mixed with the mortar used to make the first bricks. Impregnating the structure with a scent was believed to purify the site and ward off evil spirits.

The burning of incense in religious ceremony had more than one purpose in the ancient world. As well as honouring the god or goddess to whom a particular temple belonged, ancient societies also burnt incense in order to communicate with their deities. The fragrant smoke wafted upwards and literally formed a connection between the people and their gods. In fact, incense was seen very much as a two-way street. People believed that while they endeavoured to speak to the gods, the gods in turn spoke to them through that scent. They also thought that the gods themselves emitted fragrance and even fed on perfume. Likewise, the presence of a perfume was regarded as evidence of the god or goddess being there among the people.

These ideas do not disappear completely even when we move away from the pantheistic religious beliefs of these Bronze Age societies. Burning fragrant woods and resins as a means of communicating with and honouring the divine carried over into classical Greek and Roman cultures, and from there into the new religion of Christianity. The Old Testament in particular, written at different times between about 1200 BC and 165 BC, retains similar ideas about burning fragrant resins and bark as a means by which the prayers of the faithful are offered to, and heard by, God. Today, the burning of incense remains integral to the rituals and ceremonies of the Catholic Church as well as both the High Episcopal and Greek Orthodox churches.

## Scent: Health and Hygiene

In our modern world we understand that practising basic hygiene aids good health. Our bodies generally smell better for it too. We also know that certain plants have some therapeutic properties that often relate to their smell. The peoples of the Bronze Age also recognised and understood this. Scent was important to them, both in terms of keeping clean and in preventing and treating disease. Indeed, with little else to help them combat ill health, the Sumerians, Minoans, Mycenaeans and others relied on the efficacious properties of plants not only to rid them of ailments and prevent the spread of disease within their communities, but also to cover up any pervading odour of sickness.

In the ancient world, a medicinal aromatic could be applied to the skin in the form of a paste or oil, consumed with food or drink, or spread through the air to fumigate the rooms of the infirm. The sweet smell of saffron, safflower or cedarwood, for example, was used to mask the stench of putrefying limbs. One cuneiform tablet prescribes a drink made from washed raisins mixed with sixteen other ingredients including the sweet-smelling myrrh, myrtle, sweet reed, cypress and juniper as a treatment for someone suffering from a lung complaint. Perfumed oils were also widely used in gynaecological medicine in the ancient world.

Scent was used not only to treat physical illnesses but also to improve one's mental health. According to the first-century philosopher and biographer Plutarch (AD 46–119), the Ancient Egyptian perfume known as kyphi could 'lull to sleep, allay anxieties and brighten dreams'. To all intents and purposes, in the ancient world, the distinction between a scent and a medicine was non-existent. That very close connection would hold for many centuries to come.

## The Fragrance of Beauty

Perfume had yet another crucial function alongside the part it played in religious worship and maintaining health, and it is one with which we are much more familiar in our modern world: making oneself attractive to others.

Scent is a key element in the descriptions of the gods and goddesses of the ancient world who represent male and female bodily perfection. Erotic images decorate perfume containers from Antiquity, and scent as a means of seduction forms part of the erotic and sensuous bedroom scenes in ancient literature. Among the Sumerian clay tablets we find perhaps the earliest examples of erotic verse in which perfume played a key role. In one text, Inanna, the Mesopotamian goddess of love and beauty, speaks to the king. 'She called to the king: "The bed is ready!" She called to her bridegroom: "The bed is waiting!" He put his hand in her hand. He put his hand to her heart ... Inanna spoke ... "I perfumed my sides with ointment; I coated my mouth with sweet-smelling amber."'

Although men are not generally depicted beautifying themselves, scent, like make-up, is also very much part of toilette scenes in ancient art, reminding us of the part fragrance played in the beauty routines of real women in the ancient world, whose aim was to match the goddesses in all aspects of their appearance.

## The Composition of Bronze Age Fragrances: An Overview

In the past, perfume could take the form of an oily liquid, an ointment or paste or perhaps a dry powder. The finished fragrance was produced by following a lengthy method of preparation that could involve processes such as grinding, pressing and hot or cold steeping. To produce a useable amount of scent, aromatic plant material was steeped in either cold or hot oil; these methods are known respectively as maceration and enfleurage. Regardless of whichever of these processes was used, the base oil would take on the fragrance of the plant or plants in which it had been soaked. The ancients also included a resin (or perhaps honey) both to fix the scent and to add texture to the finished product. A red or reddish-brown dye extracted from the leaves of the henna tree or the roots of the herb alkanet could be added to give some colour and to make the finished product look more appealing.

Making a scent was undoubtedly a time-consuming business. In the first place, it was necessary to collect vast amounts of raw material to create an inordinately small amount of fragrant oil. Secondly, the manufacture of the finished perfume almost certainly required repeated steeping or boiling of the mixture to produce the end the result. This made for a long-drawn-out process.

The most common types of aromatic in use at this time included various kinds of woods, resins and herbs; for example cedarwood, sandalwood, terebinth resin, beeswax, coriander and fennel. Sage, cassia, rose, cinnamon, artemisia, marjoram, iris, juniper, and of course frankincense and myrrh are known from this period too. We find evidence for collection of saffron, an expensive spice used in perfume, in frescoes at the Minoan palace at Knossos on the island of Crete.

Not all these materials were available locally to those who wished to make use of them. To satisfy demand, the Bronze Age peoples traded with each other across sea and land as well as doing business more indirectly with caravans from Arabia and even China. Spices such as cassia from China and frankincense from southern Arabia found their way along the Spice Routes (largely by sea) and along the Silk Road (a land route) into the Near East and the Mediterranean. Shepherds on Crete collected a gum resin called labdanum, otherwise known as the rock rose, with a rake-like instrument. This was an aromatic, sticky material that clung to the beards of their grazing goats. What they did not need they sold on to traders for use in making perfumes elsewhere.

## The Sumerians and Babylonians

> To the god Marduk [patron deity of the city of Babylon] I anoint myself everyday with oil, burn perfumes and use cosmetics that make me worthier of worshipping thee.
>
> Nebuchadnezzar II (*c.* 642 BC–562 BC)

To the Sumerians and Babylonians perfume was a highly valued commodity. The quality of their perfumes is not in doubt, but the ingredients are sometimes hard to identify. Cuneiform tablets can be quite vague as to the specific aromatics to which they refer, noting for example 'fine oil of grand trees' or 'fine oil of some aromas'. However, even some of the oldest tablets, which date from 2100 BC, refer to myrtle, asafoetida, thyme and willow bark. Cedar, cypress, juniper, myrtle and possibly calamus and apricot were also used in the making of scent at this time. If difficulty in identifying particular plants is one problem, then the fact that the cuneiform tablets do not give much detail on proportions of ingredients is another. As a result, it is difficult for us to replicate these fragrances today.

The writing on the tablets often comprises financial accounts so, as one might expect, they tend to concentrate on prices. However, where recipes are given, there is considerable detail about the method of production, whether it is grinding, pressing, macerating, heating and filtering or a combination thereof. The cuneiform tablets are also a source of information relating to prescriptions for medical treatments which often involve the use of scents such as cassia, myrtle or asafoetida. Incidentally, willow bark, referred to in the oldest of the cuneiform tablets, contains salicin, a chemical which forms the basis of modern aspirin – the Latin word *salix* means willow.

Typically scent had a range of formal and ritually significant uses for these people too. Army commanders could be anointed with perfume before battle. Scent might be offered in tribute or given as a diplomatic gift. Perfumed textiles were presented as offerings to the gods. The *Epic of Gilgamesh*, a lengthy poem from ancient Mesopotamia (and first written down on twelve cuneiform tablets in the seventh century BC), contains a version of the biblical ark and the flood story in the context of which fragrant plants are offered to the gods who are then attracted by the scent. Utanapistim, a survivor of the great flood whose story mirrors that of Noah, says:

> I brought out an offering and offered in four directions I set up an incense offering on the summit of the mountain, I arranged seven and seven cult vessels, I heaped reeds, cedar and myrtle in their perfume burners. The gods smelled the savour; the gods smelled the sweet savour, the gods crowded round the sacrificer like flies.

The Sumerians and Babylonians used scent to anoint their statues and the walls of sacred buildings. Dead bodies were sprinkled with perfume as an act of purification. This was a practical measure as well as a religious ritual in that the pleasant smell masked the odour of death. The horns of animals for sacrifice were anointed with perfumed oil and such horns were also used as containers for sacrificial oil. This practice is evidenced at the Bronze Age site of Urkesh (in the foothills of the Taurus Mountains), a Syrio-Mesopotamian city state which flourished around 2250 BC. The raw materials used as incense inside the temples included cedar, cypress, juniper and boxwood and the pervasive odour would have filled the senses of the people living and working in the area outside the temple as well as those involved in any activity inside.

The Sumerians and Babylonians used perfumes for pleasure too. Elite Sumerians (both men and women) coated their hair with perfumed oil to give their locks a shiny appearance. Labdanum resin may have been used to keep the sculpted beards of Sumerian upper-class men in place. Dinner guests invited to a meal in one of the royal palaces or to the home of an important member of society would be surrounded by pleasant aromas as part of the dining experience. Guests might have their feet washed with scented oils. They would almost certainly be provided with rosewater to wash their hands and offered perfumed wine to drink. These guests might be gifted jars of ointments set at their place at the dining table. Both guests and their hosts customarily donned garlands of flowers at dinner.

## Perfume and Royalty

For the Sumerian rulers, and their successors the Babylonians, the use of perfume was not only considered their right but also indicative of their divine status. We know that in law the members of the royal Babylonian family were provided with fragrant oils. Beyond the use made of it by the immediate royal family, however, the king also doled out scent to the women of his harem as he saw fit. After all, scent was an essential part of their daily beauty regime in preparation for his visits. In the ancient Mesopotamian city of Mari, records show that the king distributed juniper and cypress oil to his high-ranking officials too.

The Babylonians clearly loved scent and their lavish use of it lived long in the memory. Writing centuries later, the ancient Greek historian Herodotus (*c.* 484–*c.* 425 BC) remarked, 'They grow their hair long, wear turbans and perfume themselves all over.' Later still, this time at the beginning of the third century AD, the Greek rhetorician Athenaeus of Naucratis refers to scent when he comments on the luxurious nature of the Babylonian Empire: 'At royal banquets, when the garlands are given to the guests, some slaves come in with little pouches full of Babylonian perfumes and going round the room at a little distance from the guests they bedew their garlands with the perfumes.'

## The Perfume Makers

Two names feature on one cuneiform tablet that is believed to date from 1239 BC. The first is named Tapputi. For the other we only have part of a name: Ninu. Both are described as perfume makers at the Babylonian royal palace. No doubt because of the importance of scent as a commodity but also because of the level of skill involved in the making of perfumes, these particular individuals were high-ranking members of the royal household. However, the reader might be surprised to learn that both Tapputi and Ninu were women. Although men probably predominated in the profession, judging by the status given to Tapputi in particular it seems gender didn't have to be a barrier to success.

We know nothing about Ninu aside from part of her name and her place of work, but some details about Tapputi have survived. She is referred to as *Belatekallim*, which means 'female palace overseer'. We also know that Tapputi wrote a treatise on perfume, though it has not survived. Furthermore, she is credited as being the first recorded perfume maker to work with a still, a piece of equipment for distilling and filtering liquids. She is known to have used other methods such as enfleurage as well. Even a perfume recipe attributed to her has survived; it is a fragrant ointment made for the Babylonian King Tukulti-Ninurta I, who reigned from 1244 BC until 1208 BC, and it was composed of a mixture of oil of sweet flag or calamus together with cypress, myrrh and balsam. Alongside these ingredients, the cuneiform tablet also records the process of making the scent. Tapputi included a solvent and filtered the mixture as many as twenty times to perfect the finished product. It is easy to see why a skilled worker like Tapputi, able to manufacture a quality and highly expensive product which took time and care to make, should have held such a high status within her society.

## Bronze Age Greece: Minoan Perfume and Mycenaean Scent

> Out in the dark blue sea there lies a land called Crete, a rich and
> lovely land, washed by the waves on every side, densely peopled
> and boasting ninety cities ... One of the ninety towns is a great city
> called Knossos, and there, for nine years, King Minos ruled.
>
> Homer, *The Odyssey* (*c.* 800 BC)

The Minoan civilisation which centred on the island of Crete was at the peak of its power, influence and standard of living between the sixteenth century BC and the twelfth century BC. In fact, it was an important centre of perfume production right up until the Minoan civilisation was destroyed in an enormous volcanic eruption that took place on the nearby island of Thera (modern Santorini). Evidence of the nature, use and value of Minoan perfume comes from tablets written in Linear B as well as wall paintings and pieces of pottery. It is clear that scent continued to serve a variety of practical purposes and seems to have been more widely used across Minoan society than it had been in the case of the Sumerians and Babylonians, for whom it had been very much the prerogative of the rich. However, certain scents were still intended only for the use of royalty and others who held the highest positions in society; oil of iris is one example.

The Minoans favoured compound fragrances that made use of native plants such as the herbs cumin, fennel, mint, sesame and coriander as well as turpentine (a resin extracted mainly from pine trees), iris and pomegranate. We can see these plants illustrated in the frescoes painted on the walls of important buildings, in particular a depiction of the harvesting of saffron, which although odourless when freshly picked develops a scent when dried. Whether liquid, semi-liquid or solid, Minoan scent was again oil-based with the most commonly used oils being olive and terebinth. To supplement their native plants, the Minoans imported cinnamon, myrrh, henna and nard as well as balanos oil. In turn, they exported olive and almond oil and labdanum or rock rose resin. They also exported their finished perfumes. Minoan scents were particularly popular with Egyptians of the eighteenth and nineteenth dynasties, with whom the Minoans had extensive trade links.

Typically, in the case of both the Minoan and Mycenaean civilisations, these perfumes were fatty, oily perfumes that could be smeared onto the body, burnt in honour of the gods and used to freshen the air or to scent textiles and clothing. However, in contrast to the compound perfumes favoured by the Minoans, the Mycenaeans, who lived on the Greek mainland (on the southern Peloponnese), seem to have favoured perfumes based on one major ingredient. The scientific analysis of one perfume jar from the period revealed fennel as the main ingredient. Sage or rose were also popular, simple scents. However, one partially translated Linear B tablet from a property known as the House of the Oil Merchant at Mycenae specifically records a scent made from a mixture of coriander, cumin and pennyroyal.

## Perfumes and Palaces in Bronze Age Greece

The price of a scent was considerable. It could be weighed against the same scale as gold, and could cost even more. Its manufacture was so profitable and so important that production in Bronze Age Greece was controlled from the royal palaces and the finished product either held inside the palace compound or at nearby sites. Meticulously kept written records relating to perfume production have been uncovered at the Minoan palace of Knossos on Crete and at the Mycenaean royal palace at Pylos (known as the palace of Nestor) in the southern Peloponnese. There is evidence (material and written) for the manufacture of scent at the smaller and less well-known palace of Zakros on the eastern coast of Crete too.

In the case of the palace of Nestor, the evidence points to some of the initial processing taking place in and around Pylos – that is, outside the palace – perhaps in order not to disrupt the lavish lifestyles of those who lived there and to accommodate the apparatus needed for manufacture. However, a certain amount of the manufacturing process was carried out within the palace itself. Large vats have been discovered at the north-western end of the main building.

Among the skilled artisans working to produce these perfumes at Pylos, four of them are known to us by name. One was Thyestes, which in early Greek means 'the unguent boiler'; perhaps not so much of a name as a designation, then. One clay tablet reads, 'Akosotas gave to Thyestes the unguent boiler aromatics for unguent destined for boiling.' The text goes on to list coriander, cyperus, fruits (unspecified), wine, honey, wool and must or grape juice. Unfortunately, although amounts are given, we don't know how much finished product these ingredients would have made or how long the supply was intended to last, which makes it difficult to put this information in context. Recent research does suggest the quantities are quite large, though perhaps not quite enough for a whole year's supply.

While some of the Thyestes text is inevitably difficult to interpret, it is possible to attempt some understanding. The fruits referred to might be apple or quince, and we know that wine was used to make perfume in ancient Greece while honey was added to thicken the mixture. While the mention of wool might seem curious at first, it may be that lanolin was extracted from wool for use as a fatty base for the scent, particularly as no other base oil is mentioned. Another possibility is that the base oil was supplied separately and the wool was used to strain scented oil, a technique still used in the modern perfume industry to remove impurities. Ironically, we know that in the ancient world fragrance was added to spindle wool to disguise the smell of lanolin; natural wool in itself does not have a particularly pleasant smell.

Archaeologists discovered a cluster of perfume workshops in the southern wing of the smaller palace of Zakros on Crete. An impressive vat for mixing perfumes was also found there along with large storage vessels for oil known as *pithoi*. Vessels like these have been excavated at a number of sites, notably at Mochlos, an outpost of the Minoan civilisation on the eastern side of Crete. The artisans working at Mochlos were connected with the palace administration at Knossos, where perfume processing was carried out within the palace.

That large-scale perfume production took place at all these Bronze Age palace sites is clear not only from the range of artefacts and equipment discovered there but also from the meticulous records kept by the many scribes employed in the industry. Each scribe was given very specific tasks, among them ordering the raw ingredients, taking inventory of stocks and recording the sale and distribution of the finished products. The space, time and manpower devoted to the perfume industry as well as the fact that it was under direct control of those at the very pinnacle of the social scale is an indication of its importance economically and socially. In political and personal terms, the king's grasp on the production of perfume was evidence of his power.

## Bronze Age Perfume Factories

Chamalevri on the western side of the island of Crete was producing aromatics before 2000 BC, but possibly the earliest evidence for commercial production in what we might call a factory setting comes from around that time at the site at Pyrgos, a village to the east of the tourist resort of Limassol on Cyprus. We can call it a factory because of the scale of production that went on there and because, unlike previous examples, the site was not a royal residence. Nor was perfume the only thing manufactured here; there was also work to produce copper, wine, medicines, cosmetics, textiles and olive oil.

At Pyrgos the plants used to make perfume were mostly locally grown. In fact, archaeologists have uncovered evidence for the presence of at least fourteen different native plants at this site. They include coriander, bergamot, laurel, myrtle, lavender and rosemary. Bottles, jugs and funnels used in the manufacture of perfume have also been found, as has the earliest physical example of a perfume still. Archaeological discoveries such as this, along with other clues like the reference to a still being used by our perfumer Tapputi, reveal that the process of distilling was a known means of making perfumes at this time, if not widely used; it was previously thought that the Arabs invented this method of production much later, in the seventh century AD.

The factory at Pyrgos was destroyed in 1850 BC by the earthquake on the island of Thera that wiped out the entire Minoan civilisation. No doubt the volatile oils used in perfume production there helped to fan the flames of fires that would have broken out during the earthquake. On a more positive note, from our point of view, the intense heat this generated was probably responsible for traces of the perfume industry remaining there for modern archaeologists to examine; ancient perfumes have been recreated from remnants in vessels found at the site.

## Packaging and Preservation

As well as being of great value, perfumes in Antiquity were by their very nature fragile and volatile. Therefore, in order that these precious scents could be preserved in their best condition for as long as possible, the choice of containers used for transport and storage was very important. For ancient peoples, without the synthetic fixatives available to modern-day perfumers, this was no small challenge. In the Bronze Age, perfume containers tended to be made from dense materials including hard mineral or bone such as alabaster, calcite (a common mineral which was easy to mould), porphyry (an igneous rock speckled with crystals) or ivory. All of these materials are non-porous, which would have helped to keep the contents cool and preserve the precious fragrance within.

Different sizes of vessel were used to transport and then to dispense these fragrances. Larger jars such as stirrup jars (so called because of the shape of their handles) were deemed suitable for transporting scented oils in large quantities. The stirrup jar had a narrow neck that allowed liquid or semi-liquid to be decanted sparingly, and examples have been found at the sites of palaces, temples and households. The Canaanite amphora, a two-handled jar with a pointed base suited to being stacked or lodged in soft ground, was another type of large storage container intended for transporting goods over long distances. Canaanite amphorae containing terebinth resin were retrieved from remains of the Uluburun Shipwreck, which dates from the late Bronze Age and was found off the coast of south-western Turkey; terebinth resin was a key ingredient in Bronze Age scents, especially incense. Perfume, or at least some of the ingredients required to make it, was clearly part of this ship's cargo.

Once the batch of scent reached its destination the contents of these large containers would be poured into smaller vessels, which were then quickly stoppered and sealed. When it came to the finished product, depending on how the perfume was to be used, these smaller vessels might be shaped so that the contents could be dispensed all at once, or alternatively the vessel would have a more dropper-like aperture which would allow the perfume to be released slowly and in small amounts. A perfume that was to be used as a one-off – as a libation at a funeral, perhaps – would be poured from a vessel that allowed all the contents out fairly quickly. If the scent was to be used more than once, for instance as a regular part of a lady's toilette, then a smaller amount would be needed and the shape of the container would be correspondingly different.

The variety of styles of bottles, jars, jugs and pots produced to hold scent were not only influenced by how the contents might be used, nor were they simply designed to protect the fragrance from deteriorating. The choice of vessel might also reflect the value of its contents and, in turn, the status of the owner. It is even possible that in some instances the shape of the bottle was an indication of what sort of scent was inside in a sort of early marketing ploy, though it is difficult to push this theory too far given vessels were often reused. However, there are containers with images of plants – myrtle, or the rather mysterious and unidentified silphium, for example – painted on the outside. Surely this is intended to help identify the contents within. Whatever the type of perfume they held, suffice to say for us today, these vessels are not only important finds historically speaking; many have value as works of art in their own right.

## Ancient Egypt

In the early history of Ancient Egypt, scent in all its forms was reserved only for the pharaohs and their families and those who belonged to the highest ranks in Egyptian society such as high priests and top government officials. However, in the later period of Ancient Egyptian civilisation referred to as the New Kingdom – from around 1550 BC to 1100 BC – men and women at all levels of society seem to have made some use of scent.

Our evidence relating to perfume comes from medical papyri that record scents for healing purposes. We also find recipes and details of manufacturing methods written in hieroglyphs on the walls of various ancient Egyptian temples, in particular at Edfu on the west bank of the Nile and Philae on the island of Aswan. Both of these temples have 'perfume rooms' where the walls are adorned with inscriptions explaining in detail how to prepare the perfumes of the past. These recipes would have been seen and read by the priests of the inner sanctum, who would then have prepared the scent in accordance with the recipe. Few in Ancient Egypt would have known the exact method; the ingredients and quantities that made up the special fragrances central to these temples would have been privileged information. Alongside the perfume recipes found written on temple walls the Ancient Egyptians also inscribed curses to protect this precious data, underlining the value that contemporary society placed on perfume as a desirable commodity of both religious and secular importance.

Aside from papyri and wall inscriptions there is also a wealth of archaeological evidence relating to perfume use in ancient

Egypt. Scent containers are regularly found in the pyramids of the pharaohs and also in the tombs of other members of the ruling family, members of the priesthood and other important persons. Sometimes vessels containing expensive scents such as cinnamon appear to have been recycled or exchanged for other goods with the priests from the temples. As a result, these vessels are also found in private houses where their contents may have been used as medicines.

Traditionally, in the Old and Middle Kingdoms, the Ancient Egyptians made perfume boxes and jars from mineral or rock such as alabaster and calcite (sometimes called Egyptian alabaster). They also crafted containers from another mineral deposit called anhydrite, which was particularly popular for small scent containers as it had an attractive sheen to it and came in white, rose-pink and blue varieties. These containers were often fashioned in the shape of animals: ducks or cats, for example. From the time of the New Kingdom perfume vessels could also be made of glass. Given that archaeologists have often remarked upon the brief whiff of scent when opening a tomb for the first time, the Ancient Egyptians were pretty successful in their choice of vessels for preserving fragrances.

## Ingredients in Ancient Egyptian Scent

The Ancient Egyptians favoured compound perfumes – that is, scents made from a number of different ingredients blended together. They extracted the fragrant ingredients from plants or fruits rather than animal excreta, and steeped these ingredients in a fatty oil to form a solid perfume. The fats used by the Ancient Egyptians as a base would have been olive or almond oil or basic animal fat. They used moringa oil from the seeds of the moringa tree too. Also known as ben oil, moringa oil proved particularly useful as it did not spoil for several years. The Ancient Greeks and Romans would make use of it too, and the modern perfume industry still values it as an effective scent preservative.

While scented mixtures could be burnt on charcoal as incense, they could also be applied to the body and hair in the form of fragranced oil (for therapeutic purposes as well as a means of adornment) and, in a semi solid state, chewed and swallowed to sweeten the breath. The Ancient Egyptians prepared incense (the word in ancient Egyptian is *ntyw*) from aromatic resins, oils or fats, mixed with fruit paste made from raisins or sycamore figs. Incense often came in the shape of pastilles or round balls. The resins used included precious balsam sourced from Judea, benzoin, mastic and pistachio resin. Cinnamon and cassia (both wood bark), myrrh and frankincense (resins), and cardamom (a spice made using the seeds of plants from the ginger family) were among the possible fragrances that could be added. Other favoured scents included the blue lotus (or water lily), iris, henna, juniper, marjoram, mint, myrtle, sweet flag, and cyperus. Roses appear to be relatively rare in Egyptian perfumes, though rose garlands have been found in tombs.

## Queen Hatshepsut and the Expedition to Punt

Two particularly valuable and important resins, namely frankincense and myrrh, were much favoured by the Ancient Egyptians. The plants from which they are derived did not grow in Egypt itself but were purchased in large quantities by the Ancient Egyptians from, among others, Phoenician sea traders. However, the Ancient Egyptians also acquired these precious commodities directly for themselves. Wall paintings in the tomb of Hatshepsut, an incredibly powerful female pharaoh who ruled Egypt between 1473 BC and 1458 BC, at Deir el-Bahri on the west bank of the Nile show the large bags of frankincense which the queen brought back from her expeditions to Punt, which is probably Somalia today. Living myrrh trees are depicted in the same fresco, their roots supported in large, sturdy bags. These were planted in the gardens surrounding her tomb. The inscription that accompanies the images describes the luxury goods in detail:

The loading of the ships very heavily with marvels of the country of Punt; all goodly fragrant woods of God's Land, heaps of myrrh-resin, with fresh myrrh trees, with ebony and pure ivory, with green gold of Emu, with cinnamon wood, Khesyt wood, with Ihmut-incense, sonter-incense, eye cosmetic, with apes, monkeys, dogs, and with skins of the southern panther. Never was brought the like of this for any king who has been since the beginning.

## Health and Hygiene

The link between perfume, health and wellbeing was as firmly established in Ancient Egyptian society as it was in other Bronze Age cultures. That is to say, the Egyptians appreciated scented plants and minerals not only for their pleasant aroma but also for their therapeutic benefits. Myrrh, fennel, frankincense, cassia, thyme and juniper are among the fragrant plants used in medicines as well as in perfumes. Scent helped to counteract the hot and dry climate, providing a useful deodorant in a society where personal hygiene was very important at all levels of society.

The juices from some fruits mixed with resin and other spices such as cinnamon were also applied as a deodorant. Dried iris flower was one ingredient in ancient Egyptian dentifrices (toothpastes). Egyptians often went barefoot so they massaged their feet with perfumed oils to soften the skin and as an insect repellent. They were aware that although both myrrh and frankincense resins might be used simply for pleasure, they could also be applied as salves for healing wounds. Perfumes could help wounds pucker and heal as well as stop bleeding, deterring infection. Scent with honey and later alcohol became an antiseptic. Perfumes might be drunk as a cure for disease too.

## Perfume and the Gods

Such was the importance of perfume that there seems to have been an Egyptian god overseeing not only its manufacture but also the various uses to which fragrances might be put. Nefertem, with his lotus flower headdress, was regarded as the god with responsibility for incense. He also used the power of scent to heal. Meret, the goddess of celebration, was connected with fragrant unguents, presumably because these had a prominent role at banquets and other festivities. The god Shezmu took care of the actual manufacture of perfume along with Bast, the mother of Nefertem. In Egyptian religion the goddess Bast takes the form of a cat. Among the stylish anthropomorphic vessels found in Ancient Egyptian tombs and used to hold scent, many are in the shape of a cat. Statues of the god Nefertem have been found in tombs too; among the recently discovered stacked coffins at Saqqara (just south of modern-day Cairo), archaeologists found a statue of the god with the name of its owner, the priest Badi-Amon, etched on the base.

The gods of Ancient Egypt were connected with scent in the minds of the people in more ways than one, just as they were in other early societies. Like other Bronze Age civilisations, the Ancient Egyptians believed that fragrance not only allowed them to communicate with their many gods but also that perfume both emanated from and sustained their gods too. However, Ancient Egyptian religion was more specific on this point. According to inscriptions on temple walls, scent might derive from 'the divine limbs' and 'the spittle' of the gods. The Egyptians also believed that perfume came from the eyes, ears and skin of particular divine beings. For example, perfume was believed to be the sweat of the God Ra and, according to a recipe on the wall of the temple at Edfu, the best myrrh 'springs from the eye of Ra'. Ben oil was said to come from the eye of Horus, and lesser grades of resin were believed to come from the eyes of Thoth and Osiris and from the back of Horus.

Not only did the gods themselves smell pleasant and, according to Ancient Egyptians, exude perfume from particular parts of their bodies, but they also appreciated the scent of perfume burnt as incense in their temples in homage to them. Pharaoh Thutmose III (1479–1425 BC) is known to have imported large amounts of terebinth resin every year to be burned as incense at religious ceremonies. The Ancient Egyptians believed that the fragrant plume of smoke that arose from the burning incense awakened the gods and allowed them to make a spiritual connection, bordering on a physical link, with specific deities. Offerings of aromatics were made before the statues of the gods and goddesses in the home as well as in public places of worship on a daily basis. At Heliopolis, the centre for the worship of the sun god Helios, the Ancient Egyptian priests burnt incense three times a day.

In temple precincts, statues of deities, and in particular their eyes and the mouths, were daubed with perfumed oil. Wall paintings record ceremonies where participants were anointed with perfumed oil. The format of the ritual was strictly followed. The scent vessel was held straight out in the bearer's right hand while the incense was tossed in with the left. It is notable that resins such as frankincense contain terpenes (specific aromatic compounds) which are found in large concentrations in cannabis oil. While burning frankincense is not a strong narcotic, the smoke would probably have some psychoactive effect; enough to induce a feeling of mild euphoria, perhaps, and give the priests at worship a sense of being in a higher state of consciousness. For ritual purposes myrrh was a favourite with the Ancient Egyptians. The Book of the Dead, which is in fact not so much a book as a series of scrolls relating to Ancient Egyptian funerary practices, states that myrrh was an essential feature of the 'opening of the mouth' ceremony, a ritual performed to allow the dead to continue into the afterlife. A complex perfume called kyphi, a scent containing at least sixteen different and often expensive ingredients, was also used extensively in religious ceremonies.

Although perfume played a part in celebrations where there was less risk of unpleasant odours taking hold, as always, one of its principal functions was to mask bad smells. To cover up the smell of dying animals or decaying human flesh is one obvious reason for the use of perfume in rituals involving sacrifices or at funerals.

Oxen stuffed with frankincense or myrrh were sacrificed to Isis as a practical measure to sweeten the area as the carcass burned while also honouring the divine beings. According to the Book of the Dead, an individual must not speak to gods or those in the afterlife unless he or she is clean, dressed in fresh clothes, shod in white sandals painted with eye-paint and anointed with the finest oil of myrrh. It is clear that perfume was deeply important to every aspect of religious ceremony, funeral or otherwise, and a must for all the participants.

## Mummification: Preparing the Dead

Fragrant herbs and flowers played an important part when it came to the preservation or embalming of the dead. How the deceased was preserved depended on their wealth and status. The greater the individual, the more lavish and expensive the scents used to pack the body and the more ornate and numerable the containers left in the tomb for use in the afterlife. The actual process of mummification took about seventy days and the part aromatics played in this process was twofold. First of all, spices along with palm wine were used to clean out the body once the internal organs (except for the heart) had been removed. Once the body had been dried out it was ready for a certain amount of restoration, which was the second part of the process. The body would be stuffed with fragrant flowers and herbs not only to counter any smell but also to protect it from any encroaching bacterial destruction. The linen bands which bound the mummy might also contain fragrant plants such as myrrh, cassia and camphor oil. Not only did these fragrances help to prevent decay and preserve the body in a more lifelike state, but their use in the burial rituals also played into the Ancient Egyptian belief that a pleasant smell was related to holiness.

In one of the newest revelations about the mummification process researchers examining a papyrus known as the Papyrus Louvre-Carlsberg manuscript found that the text includes a list of aromatic ingredients and resins used by embalmers to coat a piece of red linen. The linen was placed over the face of the corpse to protect it and to repel insects. As it has only recently been examined, the actual content of the papyrus has yet to be published. It does, however, explain more clearly the function of the squares of red linen cloth that have been found in association with Egyptian mummies elsewhere.

## Flower Power: The Blue Lotus

The blue lotus, or *Nymphaea caerulea* to give it its proper name, was native to Ancient Egypt. The flower is not in fact a lotus at all, but a water lily that grew prolifically in the Nile waters. Sadly, it is now seriously endangered and virtually absent from the river itself. To the Ancient Egyptians, however, the plant was one of deep religious significance. Its flower was a symbol of rebirth as it followed the rising and setting of the sun, opening at sunrise and closing at dusk. Nefertem, the Ancient Egyptian god of fragrance, beautification and healing, is depicted either holding a blue lotus or wearing a headdress comprised of them. The flower has an intoxicating smell and the Egyptians thought taking an aromatic bath containing blue lotus mixed with coriander could cure a fever. The blue lotus may also be the plant that inspired Homer's tale of the lotus eaters in the *Odyssey*, in which the soporific, mild narcotic properties of the blue lotus flower are described thus:

> I was driven thence by foul winds for a space of nine days upon the sea, but on the tenth day we reached the land of the Lotus-eaters, who live on a food that comes from a kind of flower. Here we landed to take in fresh water, and our crews got their mid-day meal on the shore near the ships. When they had eaten and drunk I sent two of my company to see what manner of men the people of the place might be ... They started at once, and went about among the Lotus-eaters, who did them no hurt, but gave them to eat of the lotus, which was so delicious that those who ate of it left off caring about home.

The boy king Tutankhamen, who ruled Egypt from 1358 BC to 1340 BC and died about the age of eighteen, appears to have been buried in haste, having passed away unexpectedly, but there were still many items in his tomb that featured the important symbol of the blue lotus, including drinking cups and unguent vases. When his tomb was opened, Tutankhamen's body itself was found to be adorned with blue lotus flowers. Floral collars worn during the burial ceremony made of lotus flower petals with papyrus, faience (a glassy blue substance closely associated with immortality) and cornflower were also found strewn about his tomb.

## The Temple at Edfu: The Writing on the Wall

In a side room in the temple of Edfu, a sanctuary dedicated to the Ancient Egyptian god Horus, we find the formula for a perfume called hekenu inscribed on the eastern wall. The main ingredient of this fragrance is something described as the 'fruit of the sweet tree', which has been identified as myrobalanum (another word for ben oil or moringa oil). The recipe also lists two grades of frankincense, two resins, wood, charcoal, something referred to as 'best wine of the oasis', and water. There are other plants mentioned in the recipe but we have little clue as to their identification.

One important feature of this recipe is that it gives the exact quantities needed for each of the ingredients. The Ancient Egyptians were meticulous about the quantities of the ingredients that needed to be mixed together to produce the best scent. There is also a detailed description of the method of preparation, a process that took a whole year. This involved pounding the dry ingredients and sifting them before adding the wine. The so-called 'fruit of the sweet tree' needed to be pressed and boiled over a fire before being added to the other ingredients. The whole mixture was then boiled again and poured into a vessel. As well as requiring great skill, perfume making in the ancient world was often a lengthy process, perhaps more akin to the modern distilling of whisky.

## Banquets and Perfume Cones

While shrines to the gods existed in private homes and incense would have been burnt in a domestic setting, there were many other reasons why individuals might use a scent in their own homes, among them offering hospitality to guests. Wall paintings from the city of Thebes, the capital of Ancient Egypt from about 1570 BC to around 1069 BC, depict flowers in abundance as a feature at banquets. When mixed with wine offered at parties, the scent of the blue lotus flower may have had a tranquilising effect of the kind referred to in the passage from Homer's *Odyssey* quoted above, and no doubt this mild sense of euphoria added to the party mood. The erotic associations of scent in the context of feasting are emphasized in wall paintings that depict nude young female dancers; there would have been wild parties and lovemaking with scent playing a central role.

Egyptian men and women attending banquets and parties are often depicted wearing cones of unguent on their heads. The true existence of these cones had, until very recently, been a point of some academic discussion. Given the practical problems of wearing something like this on one's head, and taking into consideration what we know about the links between fragrance and divinity at this time, could these objects perhaps instead be symbols much like the halo in early Christian art? The lack of any physical evidence – namely an actual cone, or even large quantities of resin on the reasonably plentiful surviving examples of Egyptian wigs – backed up the argument for the cone being symbolic. However, in 2010, archaeologists excavated a burial at Amarna in the modern Egyptian province of Minya and which in ancient times was the short-lived capital of the eighteenth-dynasty pharaoh Akhenaten. The body within wore a cone on its head.

Another cone was found in 2015, providing conclusive proof of the existence of these strange and cumbersome items. Analysis of the remains indicates that the cones were probably about 10 centimetres in height and made not of fat or oil as had been previously thought but of perfumed wax. Perhaps the solid wax simply melted gently in the steamy atmosphere (literally and metaphorically speaking), exuding its perfume in the process. Suffice to say, debate continues over how and when, or even if, these were actually worn in life.

## Ancient Egyptian Kings and Queens

Heaven and earth are flooded with incense; odours are in the Great House. Mayest thou offer them to me, pure and cleansed, in order to express the ointment for the divine limbs.

A letter to the pharaoh Hatshepsut (d. 1458 BC)

Perfumes, especially prestigious ones, were fit for a king and, of course, a queen. Not only were the pharaohs lavish in their personal use of scent but they also controlled the manufacture, trading and distribution of perfume just as the elite members of other sophisticated Bronze Age societies had done The personal use of perfume on the body seems to have increased under Hatshepsut. It may be that during her reign (which began in 1478 BC) there was the opportunity for the trade in perfume to thrive because this was a relatively peaceful period in Ancient Egyptian history. It may also be because the pharaoh herself was very much a devotee of perfume. Scent was certainly an expression of Hatshepsut's power and other Ancient Egyptian royalty would follow suit in that respect. According to Athenaeus, a Greek author writing in the third century AD, Cleopatra and Nefertiti (wife of the pharaoh Akhenaten) had their living quarters filled with rose petals. However, like another well-known anecdote that describes the powerful fragrance emanating from Cleopatra's barge as it came up the Nile, the anecdote could be a later invention. Nevertheless, these stories are certainly in keeping with the lavish lifestyle of the pharaohs and as such they warrant our attention.

In death, too, a supply of scent was important to members of the Ancient Egyptian royal family. The tombs of the rulers of Ancient Egypt are full of unguent flasks, common belief holding that scent would be a necessity in the afterlife. In the tomb of Queen Hetepheres I (d. 2551 BC), mother of Khufu or Cheops, the builder of the Great Pyramid at Giza, archaeologists discovered a number of alabaster perfume bottles. A toilet box found among the queen's grave goods and reconstructed by the Cairo Museum housed eight bottles, seven of which are believed to have contained perfume.

Not to be outdone, Tutankhamen's tomb included a total of thirty-five alabaster perfume containers in an annex. It is estimated that his tomb contained as much as 350 litres of fragrant material. We can still marvel at the design of these bottles, though their contents were stolen long ago, scooped out by thieves who well understood their value; unlike gold, which would have to be melted down before selling, these oils could be repackaged and sold on quite easily. It is still possible to see the thieves' fingerprints on the vessels. One of the jars from Tutankhamen's tomb has been shown to contain a solid unguent identified as a mixture of animal fat and probably spikenard, a costly perfume derived from a plant belonging to the valerian family. As for the boy king himself, there was so much scented resin in the wrapping of his mummified body that he was practically glued to his coffin.

## Cleopatra and Her Perfume Factory

The famous Cleopatra, properly Cleopatra VII Philopator, has long been associated with perfume. Although she lived in the Roman period, she very much follows in the Egyptian tradition when it comes to her use and connection with perfume. A popular figure in fiction and a favourite subject of historical research, stories about Cleopatra are at best exaggerated and at worst entirely fictitious. Nevertheless, we can be certain that perfume, given her power and status, would have been an everyday necessity for the queen both privately and publicly.

It seems that the queen herself was connected with the actual manufacture of scent too. Mark Antony, Cleopatra's lover, gifted her Ein Gedi, an oasis and a long-occupied site on the western shore of the Dead Sea, having confiscated it from King Herod of Judea (72 BC–4 BC). At Ein Gedi, archaeologists have discovered evidence of large-scale perfume production including equipment, storage facilities, steeping pools and containers, indicating the employment of enfleurage or the cold steeping process of maceration. There are finds there that date from the reign of Cleopatra.

Certainly the perfumes produced here were luxury products fit for a queen. There were various grades of precious balsam including opobalsamum or balm of Gilead harvested here, as well as scented oil from a plant known as persimmon that is now extinct. Persimmon was used not only as a perfume but also as a medicine, a wine flavouring and an antidote to poisonous bites. The oil or resin flowing from the persimmon plant was a much-sought-after perfume with a long history and was used to anoint the Israelite kings. After Cleopatra's demise, the plant was harvested by the Romans.

## Famous Egyptian Perfumes

A number of Ancient Egyptian scents (as opposed to their ingredients) are known to us by name. Hekenu has already been mentioned, as has kyphi. It is probably true to say that the latter is Ancient Egypt's best-known fragrance. It is first mentioned in what scholars refer to as the Pyramid Texts of the Old Kingdom, the inscriptions on the walls and sarcophagi found at the ancient burial ground at Saqqara. The word kyphi (a Greek transcription of the ancient Egyptian word *kapet*) means 'welcome to the Gods' and refers to something being burnt, indicating the important ritual function of scent. Kyphi was most frequently burnt to please, summon and communicate with the divine. However, it could also be applied to the body for fragrance, chewed to sweeten breath, inhaled as an antidote to poison and prescribed as a treatment for asthma. It was even used as a laxative, or to promote a good night's sleep when added to wine.

The earliest surviving recipe for kyphi comes from the Ebers Papyrus, a medical text dating from approximately 1550 BC. In this text the recipe for the scent seems to have been intended for domestic use – as a medicine, and to perfume one's breath and belongings. However, its main use was as a temple incense for religious ceremonies. The more complex recipes for kyphi that appear on the temple walls at both Edfu and at Philae served this purpose. The ingredients kept secret by the priesthood in the inner sanctum of the temple included wine, honey, raisins, cinnamon, cassia, cyperus, sweet flag, cedar and juniper berries as well as resins and gums such as frankincense, myrrh, benzoin and mastic. Kyphi was particularly closely associated with the sun god Ra and burnt of an evening to ensure the safe return of the daylight and the sun the next morning.

It is likely that whatever recipe the priests followed in preparing kyphi the number of ingredients would have been a multiple of four, as the Ancient Egyptians believed that this number was significant in promoting physical health and mental wellbeing. Manetho, a priest who lived in the third century BC, wrote a treatise on the preparation of kyphi and a fragment of his writing is preserved in a work entitled *Isis and Osiris* by the later Greek philosopher and writer Plutarch (AD 46–119). According to Plutarch, 'Kyphi is a mixture of sixteen ingredients – honey, wine, raisins, cyperus [perhaps galingale], resin, myrrh, aspalathus, seselis [hartwort]; mastic, bitumen, thryon [a kind of reed or rush], dock [monk's rhubarb], as well as of both junipers (arceuthids – one called the greater, the other the less), cardamom and reed [orris-root, or root of sweet flag].' Many classical writers include recipes for kyphi and the ingredients do vary. Manetho's version, however, is as close to something contemporary as we can get.

Metopium was another notable ancient Egyptian perfume. This had a thick oil base of galbanum; the plant from which this was extracted was called metopium. Metopium was believed to be particularly useful in treating stomach ailments. The Ancient

Egyptians also valued susinum, a fragrance manufactured from large amounts of lilies mixed with myrrh and cinnamon. Balanos oil was the base for this scent. Other ingredients included the almost inevitable myrrh as well as cardamom, cinnamon and honey. The scent known as mendesium was named after the Ancient Egyptian city of Djedet: Mendes being the Latinized name for the city. Mendesium comprised a mixture of myrrh and cinnamon combined with a variety of other resins and woods. The dominant smell of samsuchinon, sacred to the crocodile god Sobek, was sweet marjoram, but again this was a compound perfume containing many other plants and resins. Clearly there was no shortage of choice in terms of perfume, though most were costly.

## The Persian Empire

Manīža scatters camphor on the bed she is preparing for her
sweetheart Bīžan and sprinkles rosewater around the bed made of
sandalwood...

Ferdowsi, *Shahnameh* (*c.* AD 977–1010)

The Persian Empire was centred on ancient Iran and flourished from the sixth century BC until around 330 BC when the empire was defeated by Alexander the Great at the Battle of Gaugamela, which is probably near Erbil in modern Iraqi Kurdistan. The Persians earned a reputation for a love of perfume. Reading the Persian poem quoted above one begins to imagine the heady combination of smells. Even the furniture gave off a scent. The Roman encyclopaedist Pliny the Elder (AD *c.* 23–79) described the Persians themselves as a race 'drenched' in perfume. Although his comments are written some centuries later and he makes much of the Persians' lavish use of scented ointments in order to criticise a lifestyle that he saw as decadent, his remarks do chime well with Ferdowsi's poem.

When it comes to particular fragrances, the Persians valued and enjoyed such scents as camphor, balsam, sandalwood, frankincense, cardamom, ben oil, musk and rose. Like other early civilisations certain perfumes were reserved for royalty and one's status might be determined by smell. Saffron was strewn in front of royal processions. In frescos, Persian rulers like Darius the Great (reigned 522 BC–486 BC) and his son and successor Xerxes (reigned 486 BC–465 BC) are shown with perfume bottles. We also see Darius and Xerxes depicted in relief with plants used in the making of perfume such as lily of the valley and the narcissus plant.

According to the Greek historian Herodotus, when Xerxes wanted to pass safely through the Hellespont, the narrow strait that links the Aegean Sea with the Sea of Marmara (now known as the Dardanelles), the king had his troops burn 'various kinds of sweet-smelling materials on the bridge and branches of myrtle were scattered on it ... Everybody was crowned with flowers.' This was all done in order to get the gods on Xerxes' side and ensure a successful outcome. Again, the truth of the story is unknown as Herodotus was writing his history somewhat after the event, but nevertheless the anecdote is in keeping with what we know about the appreciation of scent in Persia and other pre-classical civilisations.

The heavy defeat of Darius II (reigned 336 BC–330 BC) at the hands of Alexander the Great at the Battle of Issus in 333 BC signalled the beginning of the end for the Persian Empire. Following the battle, Alexander raided Darius' camp. He is said to have captured forty perfumers whom the king had employed as part of his baggage train. Alexander also captured sixty-six garland makers, whom he put to work making perfumed headgear for festivals and banquets. Accounts of the battle's aftermath also mention a bath with golden perfume jars smelling of spices and perfumes. The quality of the containers was no doubt in keeping with their contents, but there is no further detail to enlighten us.

As to Alexander the Great himself, the Roman biographer Plutarch in his *Lives of the Noble Greeks and Romans*, written some 400 years after Alexander's death, notes that the conqueror's skin exuded 'a most agreeable odour' and that 'his breath and body all over was so fragrant as to perfume the clothes which he wore.' Plutarch's remarks are intended to indicate Alexander's semi-divine status. Whether he naturally smelled good or not, especially after conquering the Persians, he did take an interest in perfumes. And his conquests facilitated the flourishing of a trade in fragrances such as sandalwood, cinnamon, spikenard, benzoin and costus. He also saw the introduction of the first animal ingredients used in perfume, including musk extracted from the anal glands of the male musk deer; this ingredient in particular would stand the test of time.

## Biblical Scent

> Take the following fine spices: 500 shekels of liquid myrrh, half
> as much (that is, 250 shekels) of fragrant cinnamon, 250 shekels
> of fragrant calamus, 500 shekels of cassia – all according to the
> sanctuary shekel – and a hin [*sic*] of olive oil. Make these into
> sacred anointing oil, a fragrant blend, the work of a perfumer.
> It will be the sacred anointing oil. Then use it to anoint the tent of
> meeting, the Ark of the Covenant law, the table and all its articles,
> the lampstand and its accessories, the altar of incense, the altar
> of burnt offering and all its utensils, and the basin with its stand.
> You shall consecrate them so they will be most holy, and whatever
> touches them will be holy.
>
> Exodus 30:23–29

According to the Bible, the words above are the divine instructions given to Moses so that he could create incense to use in holy worship of Yahweh, the Hebrew name for God. Written between 1200 and 165 BC, the Old Testament makes numerous references to scent, demonstrating just how important fragrance was to everyday life not only in the context of worship but also in cleanliness (especially feminine purity), adornment and pleasure, particularly of the sexual variety. Indeed, the Old Testament does not shy away from this last topic.

As well as the fragrances used in the sacred anointing oil noted above, the Bible mentions many others more than once. These include hyssop, coriander, juniper, myrtle, spikenard, nard, cinnamon, Balm of Judea and valerian. Noah burns cedar wood and myrrh to give thanks for surviving the flood. The Book of Esther mentions breath fresheners and the sprinkling of furniture and bed linen with perfume.

In the Song of Songs, which is essentially a wedding hymn – or, to give it is proper name, an epithalamium – the writer exploits the sensual properties of fragrance, using it as a motif for both ritual and sexual attraction. The woman says to the man, 'You are fragrant, you are myrrh and aloes. All the young women want you.' In the formal praise-song in which she scrutinizes his body, moving her gaze from his head to his feet, her attention lingers on 'his cheeks a bed of spices/a treasure of precious scents, his lips/red lilies wet with myrrh'. Reading the Song of Songs, perfume predominates in a very secular way. The book is almost a catalogue of scented plants: 'Spikenard and saffron, sweet cane and cinnamon with every incense bearing tree myrrh and aloes.'

Again, in the story of Judith and Holofernes, the purpose of perfume is seduction and so it is in the story of Ruth and Boaz: 'Wash, perfume yourself and put on your best clothes.' In the Book of Proverbs we find the story of how a woman seduces an innocent young man in a bed 'perfumed with myrrh, aloes and cinnamon'. Elsewhere in the Old Testament the economic value of scent is emphasised. The Queen of Sheba brings a gift of balsam to King Solomon, a present of greater value than gold at the time – fine balsam was sold by weight at double the price of gold.

The Bible also records penalties for the misuse of perfume. In the Book of Exodus the instructions on how to make a holy incense carry a warning: 'Do not make any incense with this formula for yourselves; consider it holy to the Lord.

Whoever makes incense like it to enjoy its fragrance must be cut off from their people.' In Zoroastrianism, the probable religion of the Three Magi, fragrance was an aid to worship too. Zoroaster himself was said to have inhaled a perfume that gave him all knowledge.

Of the three gifts the Magi give to the baby Jesus, two – namely myrrh and frankincense – are expensive aromatic resins. Much has been made of the symbolic meaning of these gifts. Myrrh is believed to prefigure the death of Jesus on the cross, while frankincense is symbolic of his divine status. In the New Testament the woman in Matthew's gospel who pours valuable scented oil on Jesus' feet is criticised for doing so because of the value of the oil. Ultimately, Jesus' body is wrapped in linen cloth scented with spices. While there is no doubt that symbolic meaning exists in the stories surrounding the death of Jesus, these mentions of scent are also grounded in reality as aromatics were a normal part of contemporary burial ritual.

## The Etruscans: Italy before Rome

The Etruscans, who inhabited central Italy from around 700 BC until the first century BC, valued fragrance too. One of their gods is named Lasa and is a spirit of adornment, the Etruscan equivalent of the Greek Aphrodite or Roman Venus. Also a goddess of fate, Lasa is depicted as a naked winged female figure often carrying a perfume bottle. She appears on mirrors and among grave goods. Lasa was one of the handmaids of Turan, the Etruscan goddess of love.

Unguent jars found in Etruscan tombs commonly take the form of birds or animal shapes. A pin or dipstick was used to extract the contents, which were in a semi-solid state; kaolin was used to thicken the mixture. The Etruscans used these perfume dippers or pins, made of bronze or ivory, to apply perfume to their hair and to their bodies. The toilette box or *cista* would have stored a perfume bottle or bottles alongside a lady's mirror, comb and pins. These boxes were made of bronze with a handle formed usually in the shape of two figures. A cream found at the important Etruscan town of Chuisi among the grave contents of a wealthy Etruscan lady is an excellent example of a perfumed product geographically distanced from its original origin, in this case Egypt, being used by a member of the early Italian élite. On account of the good state of preservation, analysis was able to reveal that the cream may have been used simply as a perfume or perhaps a skin softener as it consisted of moringa oil and two plant resins, namely mastic and pine.

# 3

## THE CLASSICAL WORLD
### Scent in Myth and in Reality in Ancient Greece and Rome

[Aphrodite] passed into her sweet-smelling temple. There she went
in and put to the glittering doors, and there the Graces bathed
her with heavenly oil such as blooms upon the bodies of the
eternal gods – oil divinely sweet, which she had by her, filled with
fragrance.

'To Aphrodite', *Homeric Hymns* (*c.* 700–600 BC)

For the Greeks and Romans, the very origins of scent were shrouded in myth and legend. Among the deities of the classical world the Greek goddess Aphrodite established herself not only as the goddess of love and beauty but more specifically the divinity with responsibility for perfume. According to tradition, a river nymph named Oenone obtained the secrets of perfume from Aphrodite. The name Oenone, according to the fourth-century BC grammarian Lycophron, means 'skilled with drugs'; this is appropriate given the already longstanding close association between scent and medicine. Oenone, so the story goes, passed on the secrets of scent to Paris, Prince of Troy, who betrayed Oenone with the beautiful Helen, wife of Menelaus, King of Sparta, sparking the infamous Trojan War. Helen then took her acquired knowledge of scent back home with her when she returned to Greece.

In classical legend, Aphrodite (and her Roman equivalent Venus) is bathed in sweet-smelling oils as she rises up from the sea, born in the form of a full grown and perfect woman. The goddess uses scent to enhance her own attractiveness. Fragrance is an integral part of her identity. Even her hair 'breathed out a supernatural perfume' according to the poet Virgil (70 BC–19 BC). The goddess makes use of the perceived healing power of scent too. When, in Virgil's epic poem the *Aeneid*, Aphrodite's son Aeneas is seriously hurt, the goddess 'sprinkles the liquid of healing ambrosia and sweet-scented all-heal' on the wound.

Aphrodite's attendants, the Kharites – or Graces, as they are more often called – are also closely associated with scent. According to one poem, written in the seventh century BC by an unknown author, the Graces themselves smelled of 'crocus, hyacinth, and blooming violet, and the sweet petals of the peerless rose, so fragrant, so divine'. Although the context is fictional (as far as we are concerned), we can nevertheless get a sense of the flowers known and appreciated for their scent in the real world at this time.

Other divinities, male as well as female, were also linked with fragrance. They include Zeus, the chief among the gods, who sits atop a fragrant cloud. Of Diana, goddess of the moon and hunting, the fifth-century BC Greek playwright Euripides (484 BC–406 BC) writes, 'O Diana sweet goddess I know that thou art near me for I recognised they balmy odour.' It is clear that the Greeks and Romans, just like the earlier Bronze Age civilisations, adhered to the belief that perfume was an attribute of the divine and an indication that they were in the presence of a god or goddess.

## Scent and the Image of Heaven

It was not only the Greek and Roman gods and goddesses themselves who were believed to be fragrant. Classical authors describe their dwelling place (and that of those good men and women worthy enough to live with them) as sweet smelling.

The Land of the Blessed or the Elysian Fields was the classical equivalent of heaven and its sweet fragrances were well known. In the words of the Greek historian Herodotus:

> In the Elysian Fields there is a golden city with emerald fortifications and roads paved with ivory where the gates are made of cinnamon. Around the walls the River of perfume flows one hundred cubits wide and deep enough that one could swim in it. The baths are crystal edifices held up by pillars of fragrant wood and the bathtubs a warm and pleasantly odiferous dew is ever flowing ... five hundred fountains of fine fragrance ... charming nightingales fill the air with their song and pick up fragrant blossoms which they drop in front of their guests like scented snow and a thick vapour rises from the perfumed river and floats within the banquet hall imparting a refined and suave fragrant dew.

Note how prominently scent features in this passage. This is not only a pretty illusion but a reflection, no doubt, of the degree to which contemporary society valued fragrance in real life. Indeed, many of the features described by Herodotus would be replicated in reality, becoming part of the lifestyle of the social elite of the classical world, especially at the height of the Roman Empire.

## Perfume in Everyday Life

> Let the rich fumes of odorous incense fly
> A grateful savour to the powers on high
> The due libation nor neglect to pay
> When evening closes or when breaks the day
> Hesiod, *Works and Days* (c. 700 BC)

In the context of day-to-day living in the Greek and Roman world, scent was in fact given just as much importance as it was in classical myth and legend. Contemporary authors might interpret perfume as a physical and material symbol of wealth and status and, on a more practical (and very personal) level, as a necessary component of good health, bodily attractiveness and the freshness of youth. Men and women wore perfume to counteract excessive sweating, underarm body odour and even bad breath as well as using it to protect against disease and cure its symptoms. Both applied scent as means of making themselves sexually attractive to others.

Scent fitted well into some of the well-worn themes or *topoi* of classic literature too, particularly the notion of the past as a golden age and the merits or demerits, depending on one's point of view, of city living. In his comic play *Mostellaria* (which translates as *The Haunted House*), the Roman playwright Plautus (254 BC–184 BC) introduces one of these popular themes, with urbane sophistication contrasted with the simplicity of rural life through the mouths of two slaves. Tranio, the urban slave, remarks, 'May Jupiter and all the gods destroy you! You smell strongly of garlic. Lump of native filth thick he-goat pigsty mixture of mire and manure!' Grumio, the country slave, acknowledges his comments and contrasts himself with his city counterpart: 'What do you want me to do?' He asks. 'We can't all smell of exotic perfumes.' Other authors extolled the virtues of fragrance too. The elegiac poet Ovid (43 BC–AD 17) in particular was an ardent admirer of perfumes and cosmetics too. He saw both as elements of refinement and cultured living that thrived in an urban environment.

However, while fragrance was certainly a popular theme in descriptions of everyday life, unlike its esteemed place in myth and legend the topic does not always get a good press when describing the real world in the classical period. In fact, Ovid in his fervour for all things sophisticated sometimes seems the exception rather than the rule. In contrast to him, the famous orator Cicero (106 BC–43 BC) considered the use of perfume an unnecessary extravagance. He also labelled perfume manufacture a base industry and declared with disgust that in his time even soldiers wore scented hair oil under their helmets.

He interpreted the latter as a sign of the degeneration of contemporary society from the perceived high moral standards of the past. The playwright and philosopher Seneca (*c.* 4 BC–AD 65) also saw the rougher, less pleasant smell of sweat and body odour as virtuous, reminding us that 'in the early days ... pretty dirty fellows they evidently were but they smelled of the camp, the farm and heroism.' The perpetrators of the Catiline Conspiracy of 63 BC, who sought to overthrow the consulship of Cicero and his colleague Gaius Antonius Hybrida, were alleged to have been discovered in their hiding place because of their heavy and excessive perfume. True or not, the reference to scent here gave weight to the idea that the conspirators were immoral degenerates.

Although scent was a commodity important to economic growth, particularly under the Roman Empire, even this lucrative trade in exotic plants and spices attracted some criticism, mainly for drawing money away from Rome and upsetting the balance of import and export trade. Emperor Tiberius, who ruled from AD 14 to 37, complained to the Senate about the huge amount of money that Roman citizens spent on perfume. Indeed, he claimed that their extravagance drained the economy of an enormous 100 million sestertii each year.

Alongside criticism of society in general, satirists, comedy writers and historians alike employed fragrance as a metaphorical tool to pour scorn on those belonging to particular social groups. For example, Plautus criticised older women for allegedly overusing scent to attract male attention and regain an appearance of lost youth. Seneca describes the common prostitutes who frequented the public spaces in Rome as 'saturated with drink and perfume'; according to him they had completely overdone it.

Classical authors even used scent as a tool to defame particular individuals. The emperors were certainly not immune to such criticism. The Greek philosopher Plutarch mocked Emperor Nero (who reigned from AD 54 to 68) for filling the rooms of his palace with costly perfume; however, the philosopher only dared to venture this criticism after the somewhat volatile Nero was dead. The encyclopaedist Pliny the Elder, who maintained that it was the quest for luxury that drove men to create perfumes in the first place, chastised Emperor Otho (who ruled for only a few months in AD 69) for applying perfume to the soles of his feet; to do so was a custom associated with people who were not citizens of Rome.

Much of the denigration of perfume in classical texts is pure rhetoric, employed to help the topic fit with common themes. However, whatever the thoughts of many of those who commented on perfume, their regular reference to it is in itself an indication of its prevalence and profusion in everyday classical life. We can tease out some facts even when the remarks made are negative.

## Making and Using Scent

> Perfumes are compounded from various parts of the plants:
> flowers, leaves, twigs, root, wood, fruit, and gum; and in most cases
> the perfume is made from the mixture of several parts.
>
> Theophrastus, 'On Odours'

For the Greeks and Romans, perfume (the general term in Ancient Greek was *muron* and in Latin *unguentum*) came in various forms: solid or semi-solid, liquid or powder. Their perfumes were based on vegetable oils such as olive oil, almond oil and sesame oil. The more expensive balanos oil (expressed from the kernels of a tree native to Egypt) was also an option. To this was added an astringent, such as ginger grass or aspelathus. The latter is better known to us today as rooibos, the leaves of which are used to make herbal tea. The addition of an astringent, according to contemporary sources, made the base mixture more receptive to the main ingredient – that is, the fragrance. The scents used were composed mainly of plant material. Indeed, any number of flowers, petals, seeds, leaves as well as resins could be added to impart an agreeable odour: roses, bergamot, quince blossoms, lilies, spikenard, myrrh and frankincense to name but a few. The methods used by the people of the classical period to make perfume included expression, hot or cold steeping and various methods of extraction and straining.

Scent was part of the social and cultural fabric for Greeks and Romans. Festivities such as weddings and dinner parties, as well as religious rituals, including feast days and funerals, used perfume in the form of incense and libations to the gods, and when it came to personal use it was not only women who wore perfume. The use of fragrance reached its height under the Roman Empire when the elite members of society perfumed almost everything, even the furniture and fittings in their homes including drapes, candlesticks, tables and cushions. No doubt by this time some of the criticism of the use of scent we find in Latin texts was justified: the use of scent had become excessive. If we are to believe the ancient historians, some of the more decadent emperors, including Elagabalus (reigned AD 218–222) and Nero (reigned AD 54–68), even perfumed their dogs and horses. Birds scented with perfume were released into the air at banquets so that the guests could enjoy fragrance as part of their dining experience; all this is reminiscent of Herodotus' description of the Elysian Fields, the home of the gods.

As far as Pliny the Elder was concerned, not only was there a great deal of choice when it came to scent but there were fashion trends to be taken into account as well:

> The perfume of iris, from Corinth, was long held in the highest esteem, till that of Cyzicus came into fashion. It was the same, too, with the perfume of roses, from Phaselis, the repute of which was afterwards eclipsed by those of Neapolis, Capua ... Oil of saffron, from Soli in Cilicia, was for a long time held in repute beyond any other, and then that from Rhodes; after which perfume of œnanthe from Cyprus came into fashion, and then that of Egypt was preferred. At a later period that of Adramytteum came into

vogue, and then was supplanted by unguent of marjoram, from Cos, which in its turn was superseded by quince blossom unguent from the same place.

One should not dismiss trends in perfumes as unimportant; mere fashion they may be, but they had significant economic and social implications.

## The Science of Scent: Theophrastus, Dioscurides and Pliny the Elder

Such was the importance of perfume to society that many learned men chose to write about it. Classical authors Theophrastus, Dioscurides and Pliny the Elder all made studies of perfume because they understood its significance – medically, socially and economically – to the people of the time. Greek philosopher Theophrastus (*c.* 371 BC–287 BC) was a pupil of Aristotle and eventually succeeded him as head of the Greek peripatetic school of philosophy. Theophrastus made an extensive study of plants, work that has earned him the title 'Father of Botany'. He left his knowledge to us in nine treatises entitled *Enquiry into Plants* (*Historia Plantarum*); a tenth book survived up until the Middle Ages but is now lost. In part of this work, entitled 'On Odours', he examines the importance and use of perfumes in Greek society, noting that scent was mixed into wine, used to perfume bedsheets and applied to the body; indeed, he notes that '[fragrant] powders are used for bedding, so that they may come in contact with the skin'. Theophrastus also believed that there was a strong link between taste and smell which had implications for appetite and therefore health. He imparts in detail his knowledge not only of how to make perfume but also of how to make it last:

Now the composition and preparation of perfumes aim entirely, one may say, at making odours last. That is why men make oil the vehicle of them, since it keeps a very long time and also is most convenient for use. They use spices in the making of all perfumes;

some to thicken the oil, some in order to impart their odour. The less powerful spices are used for the thickening, and then at a later stage they put the one whose odour they wish to secure. For that which is put in last always dominates even if it is in small quantity; thus if a pound of myrrh is put into a half-pint of oil, and at a later stage a third of an ounce of cinnamon is added, this small amount dominates.

Following on from Theophrastus' work, the Greek pharmacologist, botanist and physician Dioscurides (AD 40–90), who was a medic with the Roman army, wrote a five-volume work entitled *De Materia Medica* (*On Medical Material*) about which the sixth-century statesman and scholar Cassiodorus (AD 487–585) remarked, 'Above all else consult the Herbarium of Dioscorides, who described and illustrated the herbs of the fields with amazing exactness.' *De Materia Medica* gives us a clear and detailed picture of the different processes involved in making a perfume at this time:

This is a double phase process. The purpose of the first phase is to render the oil receptive to the aroma of the flowers and the leaves to be added later. An unguent is made from the roots of calamus of gorse and cyperus plants made into a paste with pestle and mortar and mixed with water or wine which is then boiled in olive oil. The oil is then sieved through a colander and let to cool off. The second phase involved steeping into the cool oil those fragrant flower petals and leaves and roots which would give the final aroma to the product. Lastly colour for decorative purposes and salt and/or spices for preservation purposes.

Pliny the Elder used much of Dioscurides' original material. While he does, on occasion, criticise the proliferation of perfume in contemporary society as luxurious excess, at the same time he gives us much in the way of practical information about the subject as well as a sense of the astonishing range of fragrances on the market. He mentions at least twenty-two varieties of perfumed oils, among them cypress, marjoram, broom, iris, spikenard, rose, myrtle, laurel, crocus, lily, juniper, almond, carnation, poppy, pine nut, coriander, aniseed, cumin, narcissus and daisy.

## Girl Power and Scent for Men

Women applying perfume is a popular subject depicted on all manner of Greek vases and Roman wall paintings. While fragrance was seen an important component of feminine beauty, among the extant writings from the classical period there is nonetheless an evident underlying fear of women using it to distract, beguile and even deceive men. This is exemplified in the only surviving work of second-century Greek novelist Achilles Tatius, a romantic novel entitled *The Adventures of Leucippe and Clitophon*, 'Everything women do is false words and actions. Even if a woman appears beautiful it is the laborious contrivance of make-up her beauty is all perfume or hair dye or potions.' Nevertheless, Aphrodite set the standard and real women sought to emulate her. Perfume is one of the tools in the goddess's armoury, an instrument of her divine power.

The idea that perfume had a potent power may stem not just from tales about Aphrodite but also from the tradition that witches in classical literature like Medea created love potions from herbs and flowers in order to entrap men. The comparison crosses into the real world if we look at instances where named characters in fiction are in fact pseudonyms for real people. For example, the witch Canidia, who appears in no less than six poems by the lyric poet Horace (65 BC–8 BC), according to the second-century commentator and grammarian Porphyrio, may be a real woman called Gratidia who sold perfumes. As it has long been understood that the ladies who appear in Roman elegiac poetry are often real women given false names to conceal their identity, Porphyrio could indeed be correct. Suffice to say that fear of a woman's power and influence (with perfume often playing some part) is an underlying theme in the work of Roman authors in particular.

So what was perfume like for the women of ancient Greece or Rome? Contemporary fashion would have been taken into account, but women would also have had to consider availability of particular scents and the price and necessary status for certain products. Theophrastus opines that the best perfumes for women are 'myrrh oil and megalion, the Egyptian sweet marjoram and spikenard for these owing to their strength and substantial character do not easily evaporate and are not easily made to disperse and a lasting perfume is what women require'. His comments seem to be made very much from the male point of view, wanting a woman who always smells appealing and is therefore sexually attractive. We know that there is a strong link between perfume and sex appeal, and the high-class call-girls of Greek and Roman society could expect to be given scent as a gift from their ardent admirers in return for favours.

Scent worn by a man simply for its own sake could draw criticism of immorality and effeminacy in the classical world, particularly among the Romans, and this might render an individual unsuitable for public office. However, in certain situations – practising athletics, for instance – to use a fragrance was considered entirely legitimate. Images of male athletes rubbing themselves with fragrant oil are frequently to be found depicted on Greek and Roman vases. Men, both Greek and Roman, could also make use of perfume without fear of disapproval when attending a dinner party or if they were doing so for the purposes of hygiene or to ward off disease.

According to contemporary sources, there were scents that suited men rather than women. Theophrastus comments, 'The lightest perfumes are rose perfume and cypros which seem best suited to men as also is lily perfume.' Martial (AD 40–104), the writer of many short poems or epigrams, considered cinnamon an everyday perfume suitable for men. However, one might sound a note of caution here as Cosmus, the perfumer who sells and maybe produces these cinnamon fragrances, appears a number of times in Martial's verses, leading one to surmise that the poet may be advertising on his friend's behalf. The poet Catullus (*c.* 84 BC–54 BC) describes the bed of his paramour Flavius as 'adorned with flowers and garlands'. Both men and women could be said to use the power of scent, then, for sexual advantage as well as for health and hygiene purposes and as an expression of their personal wealth and status in Roman and Greek society.

## Perfume Pots

The classical civilisations of Greece and Rome, much like the peoples of the Bronze Age, took interest in the containers for their perfumes. Containers used to transport, store and dispense scent came in a wide variety of shapes and sizes and could be made from different materials. Function was a key influence on the shape and size of any given vessel. Larger vessels were used for transport but when the cargo reached its destination the contents were likely to be decanted into smaller containers for sale just as had happened in the past. However, in Ancient Greece advances in technology allowed for the making of fine small vessels with tight-fitting lids, suitable for scent. This helped to preserve the precious contents inside. Also, following on from the invention of glassblowing in Syria in the first century AD, glass perfume bottles in both simple and ornamental shapes were more plentiful. Zoomorphic shapes including fish, bears and birds were popular, and decorative containers made from expensive materials were intended to impress, to emphasise the value of their contents and, in turn, boast the status of the owner.

Some containers were clearly disposable as they needed to be broken to release their contents and could not be resealed. For example, in northern Italy a number of glass vessels have been discovered in the shape of birds, and in order to get to their contents one would need to break the bird's tail. While a vessel that can only be used once might seem extravagant, there are even some perfume vases that appear so elaborate that it is doubtful that they were ever put to practical use at all. Other types of container had very narrow necks so that they only released their precious content drop by drop. These might be refilled and used again, though not always with the same scent that they originally held – there is evidence of recycling in the classical world.

Certain vessel types have become recognisable today. The alabastron was a narrow-necked vessel from which contents were removed with a thin stick; its name recalls the popularity of alabaster as a material for scent bottles thanks to its density, which trapped smells. Unguentaria, or test-tube-shaped glass bottles, small and narrowed at the neck, are common finds at domestic sites and in funeral contexts. The rather oddly shaped askos, with a handle and spout, also released its contents drop by drop and appears in a variety of contexts from toilette scenes in relief and frescos to the detritus found at graves. The small, spherical aryballos, which was used to hold scented oil, was very portable (often attached to a chain) and was a popular accessory to take to the public baths. Such vessels are sometimes recovered by archaeologists linked by their chain to a strigil, the instrument used to scrape scented oil from a person's skin in the absence of soap as we know it. The lekythos is a taller, often highly decorated vessel found at burial sites and among grave goods and was perhaps used for pouring libations of scented oils. The exaleiptron is a vessel with an inward-curving lip, ideal for preventing spillage. The name is derived from the Greek *exaleipho*, meaning 'to wash over' or 'to anoint'. Some examples of this type of vessel are very large and intended to hold a considerable amount of scented oil for use in religious ritual or as part of the celebrations at a banquet. In contrast, the pyxis, a small pot with a lid and sometimes feet, is a common feature in toilet scenes and contained cosmetic creams, scented ointments and powders.

That such vessels are often found far from their place of manufacture is testament to the extensive trade in perfume as a valued commodity during the classical period. Also, the fact that so many glass vessels believed to have held perfume have been discovered at archaeological sites across the world is an indication of just how ubiquitous these objects would have been, particularly given the fragile nature of glass itself – if so many have survived, a great deal more have not.

## Perfume, Health and Hygiene

> There is wide use in medicine of flowers and perfumes generally.
> Pliny the Elder, *Historia Naturalis*

Unpleasant smells often accompany illness. In the classical world, the natural process of aging was also interpreted as a disease and perceived as giving off a bad odour. Therefore, for the individual it was important to appear healthy not only in terms of wellbeing but as a reflection of one's position in society and also to seem youthful. Smell was very much part of that impression.

The Ancient Greeks and Romans continued to view perfumes as medicines as previous civilisations had done. They used scent to improve both their physical wellbeing and were familiar too with the benefits of flowers, herbs and spices in aiding a person's mental state. According to the early Greek poet Alexis (*c.* 375 BC–*c.* 275 BC), 'The best recipe for health is to apply sweet scents to the brain.'

In certain branches of medicine, the application or even the consumption of a perfume was a standard treatment. Scent continued to be a common ingredient in gynaecological treatments for women; remember that scent appears to have been associated with childbirth even from prehistoric times. Perfumed ointments were also used to treat everyday ailments such as stomach complaints and skin rashes that afflicted both sexes. The Greek physician Hippocrates (460 BC–370 BC), known to us as the father of modern medicine, put his faith in the therapeutic power of plants, prescribing fumigations, rubs and aromatic baths using sage, mallow and cumin among others. Hippocrates even set up scented stakes around the city of Athens in an attempt to stem an outbreak of disease (thought to be smallpox) that occurred there in 430 BC. In his wake, Galen of Pergamon (AD 129–*c.* 200), a surgeon, philosopher and physician to Emperor Marcus Aurelius, expounded the curative properties of scent too. He prescribed fragrant chewing gum as a cure for, of all things, unpleasantly smelly armpits as well as inventing the world's first cold cream scented with rosewater, which he used not only to soften the skin (its cosmetic function today) but to treat the wounds and scars of the gladiators who fought in the arena.

## Scent at the Baths

Going to the baths was a daily ritual for the Greeks and Romans. The Romans in particular built luxurious public baths and perfuming the customers was one of the services these establishments provided. When visiting the baths you might also take along your own favourite scented oil in an ampulla or aryballos (those small, round bottles with the chain attached). If you were wealthy enough, you might have a particular slave whose job it was to carry it for you. Fragranced oil would be applied before exercising and bathing as well as after taking a bath. The scented oil was then scraped off with a strigil to remove any dirt. Ointments and oils intended for this purpose were made from various plant sources including rose, quince and narcissus.

In the Greek and Roman world, private bathing was also an option. The Roman emperor Elagabalus is alleged to have taken the use of scent to the extreme, filling his swimming pools and bathtubs with essence of rose or wormwood. As early as the fourth century BC, the Greek comic poet Antiphanes (408 BC–334 BC), in a fragment preserved in the work of Athenaeus, describes a rich man taking his bath in a large golden bathtub: 'First then he applies Egyptian unguent to his feet and oil of fragrant palm to his chest his two arms and back are scented with essence of mint. Marjoram is used on hair and brow and thyme invigorates his weakened knees.' Note that different scents were applied to different parts of the body. This, alongside the fact that he uses Egyptian unguent and his bathtub is made of gold, is a fairly clear indication of the subject's luxurious lifestyle. The passage also alludes to the well-established belief that certain odours had some medical benefit – which in this instance is not unfounded. Camphor is still applied to the chest to gain relief from the common cold and the herb thyme is still believed to be efficacious as a treatment for arthritis.

## Perfume in Public: Games, Festivals and Triumphs

The Romans are renowned for the sophistication of their drainage systems, but going outside would nevertheless have been a smelly experience in towns and cities with their crowded streets. Particularly unpleasant smells would have emanated from premises such as tanning workshops and cattle markets. Markets selling fruit and vegetables also stocked meat and fish with no regular means of refrigeration – ice was so scarce that the philosopher Seneca referred to it as a luxury. On the numerous festival days, too, the smell from animal carcasses burning on open altars mixed with all these other smells must have been overwhelming.

Perfumes were worn, carried, burnt or sprinkled to counteract these bad odours. Roman ladies held small balls of amber which they rubbed every so often to give a delicate aroma as they passed through a particularly malodorous area. Perfume played more of a central role at certain events, for instance the Greek festival of Adonis. The lover of the goddess Aphrodite, Adonis was honoured with the burning of sweet incense, probably myrrh, as he, according to Greek mythology, had been born of the myrrh tree and anointed with myrrh by Aphrodite's handmaids, the Graces. Chaplets or garlands of flowers, leaves and herbs were a common sight at special events both Greek and Roman. These were worn by victors at the games and in honour of the gods at festivals. Although garlands were generally made from fresh blooms, Pliny the Elder does mention chaplets imported from India and from Thrace made of fabric mixed with nard leaves or else 'silk of many colours steeped in unguent'.

Scent was very much part of the spectacle of an athletic performance or event. Athletes in the Greek and Roman world smeared their bodies with scented oil. Olive oil was associated with Athena in her capacity as the goddess of power and strength. The scented oil applied by the competing athletes comprised a mixture of olive oil and aromatic herbs such as cedarwood or sage. There were practical reasons for applying scented oil to the body at the gymnasium or the games, too. The oil toned the muscles of the athletes and hastened recovery from injuries while at the same time promoting cleanliness and hygiene. As a bonus, their glistening bodies may have heightened the sensuous nature of the games, as well as making them difficult to grasp in sports such as wrestling.

Notably, at the Colosseum in Rome the smell of death hung heavy in the air after the slaughter of animals and people during circuses, games and theatrical performances. The foul smell would have been exacerbated by the heat of the afternoon sun. The Romans developed a sophisticated, built-in solution to this problem whereby an elaborate system of pipes sprayed the delicate scent of saffron around the seating area and down into the stadium to freshen the air.

Perfume in all its forms was a suitable gift with which to honour important persons. Artaxerxes II, King of Persia in the fifth century BC, paid honour to the Spartan Antalcidas by sending him 'his own chaplet [of flowers] dipped in perfume'. Scent also formed part of the cult of the Roman emperor, being burned, sprayed, smeared and worn as a mark of respect for him wherever he went. When the emperor Caracalla (ruled AD 198–217) visited Alexandria in AD 215, according to the contemporary historian Herodian 'clouds of perfumes and incense provided a sweet-smelling odour in the streets and the emperor was honoured with torchlight processions and with showers of flowers'. Similarly, when Nero entered the city of Rome as emperor in AD 37, the streets were strewn with saffron before him. The soldiers who took part in the triumphant return of General Titus in AD 70, having plundered the perfume manufacturing site of Ein Gedi, waved precious and fragrant persimmon plants in celebration of their military success.

## Perfume in Private

At home, especially in the dwellings of the elite citizens who inhabited the major cities of Greece and Italy, perfume had many everyday uses. As ever, scent could cover up unappealing smells. Plant oil, particularly olive oil, was standard in the many lamps used to light private houses. Aromatic herbs or floral perfumes might be added to engender a nicer smell. Perhaps this practice is best described as an early version of the modern, and nowadays just as ubiquitous, perfumed candle. In order to wash the stains out of their clothes the Greeks and Romans bleached them with urine. Clearly this did not make their clothes smell very pleasant so they used scent to counteract this too. Dyeing cloth was not without its bad smells either. The prized purple colour that lined the togas of male Roman citizens was extracted from a shellfish called the murex; its fishy smell needed to be covered.

Scent was a precious commodity in every sense, and not a drop was wasted. Leftover dregs of perfume could be made into a powder known as diapasmata, similar to a talcum powder today, and this could be sprinkled on unworn clothing to keep the fabric fresh. The wealthy stopped at nothing when it came to perfuming their private dwellings. Mint was a popular room freshener and in the homes of the rich, famous, and indeed infamous. Even the cushions and soft furnishings were sprinkled, covered or stuffed with this and other herbs and exotic spices. The emperor Nero was said to sleep on a mattress stuffed with rose petals.

## Greek Symposiums and Roman Banquets

> Be sure and have the second course quite neat
> Adorn it with all kinds of rich confections
> Perfumes and garlands aye and frankincense
> And girls to play the flute
> Athenaeus of Naucratis, *Deipnosophistae*

The Greek symposium was a forum for male intellectual discussion as well as being an eating and drinking session accompanied by music. At their meal the men would anoint themselves with perfume or perhaps don garlands made from plants like myrtle. The whole affair was rather decadent. No doubt perfume contributed to that sense of excess, reminiscent of these Ancient Egyptian banquets described in the previous chapter. Guests at the most sumptuous of dinner parties not only wore garlands but reclined on couches stuffed with rose petals – Nero's mattress, though extravagant, was not without precedent. The host would serve aromatic wines scented and flavoured with myrrh. Pliny the Elder describes this practice, remarking that 'the most renowned wines among the ancient were those that were spiced with the scent of murra'. There were, however, some alternatives to myrrh. In the later Roman Empire it became fashionable to add nard, cinnamon, cassia, ginger or frankincense to wine.

There were various reasons why the Greeks and Romans may have perfumed their wine. According to Pliny the Elder, 'people put perfume in their drink and the bitterness this produces is highly prized. By this lavishness perfumes thus gratify two senses at once.' He noted too that the scent acted as a preservative. Cicero, on the other hand, noted that adding perfume to wine simply allowed one 'to enjoy the lavish scent both inside and outside'. However, the inclusion of perfume as part of these symposia may have had an important practical purpose as far as the participants were concerned. The scent, they believed, could prevent headaches arising from overindulgence in alcohol.

The dining room in the Domus Aurea or Golden House, an ostentatious landscaped palace built in the centre of Rome by the Emperor Nero, was said to have ivory ceiling panels that opened to shower petals and perfumes on the guests below as they dined. The Roman historian Suetonius (*c.* AD 69–122) also claimed that the Golden House had a revolving dining room. All this seemed truly fantastical until relatively recently, when archaeologists discovered the mechanism for the rotating room; if that part of the story was true, perhaps there really was a ceiling that could open to spray scent.

This effusion of perfume at dinner did not find favour with everyone, of course. The fifth-century BC Greek philosopher Xenophanes, for example, disapproved of the 'garlands, saucers with perfume, perfumed wine, flowers and incense that are part of an invitation of scholars to dinner'. While he is not a fan, his comments do give us some insight into the profusion of perfume at the dinner table, especially at the symposium.

The abundance of scented flowers at dinner parties was also potentially dangerous, at least according to the *Historia Augusta*, a late Roman collection of biographies of disputed date. One anecdote describes how Emperor Elagabalus, 'in a banqueting-room with a reversible ceiling ... once overwhelmed his parasites [hangers-on] with violets and other flowers, so that some were actually smothered to death, being unable to crawl out to the top'. Whether this anecdote has any basis in truth we cannot know. The scene is captured centuries later (see p.216), by nineteenth-century American artist Lawrence Alma-Tadema.

## Scent at Weddings and Funerals

> Nor do winsome Amor (Love) [Eros] and Gratia (Grace) [Kharis] grow weary in scattering countless blossoms and cloudy perfumes [during the wedding] o'er thee [the bridegroom] and as thou holdest close-locked the snow-white limbs of thy longed-for bride. And now roses, now lilies mixed with violets dost thou receive upon thy brow, as thou shieldest the fair face of thy mistress.
>
> Statius, *c.* AD 45–96

Scent had an important part to play in the rituals surrounding marriage and death. In the lead-up to a marriage, floral crowns were given as love tokens, worn or perhaps placed on the doorstep of a beloved by their suitor. Scent was considered an appropriate gift to give to the new couple, and perfume bottles, plain or elaborate, depending on the wealth of the bride's family might form part of the dowry a bride brought with her on the occasion of their marriage.

Perfume was also used in the wedding ceremony itself. Both bride and groom would wear perfume. The chosen scent was frequently myrtle as this was a plant sacred to Aphrodite, the goddess of love – a natural choice even when many marriages (particularly among the upper classes) were arranged with a view to business interests or establishing important personal and political connections. Garlands of sweet-smelling flowers also featured in the marriage ceremony. Athenaeus gives a list of flowers suitable for garlands on special occasions such as weddings and banquets. These include violets, wallflowers, lilies, gladioli and hyacinths.

In a letter from Roman Egypt dating from the second century AD, commercial suppliers Apollonius and his partner Serapias write to their client Dionysia begging her pardon for a shortage of blooms for her wedding: 'There are not many roses here – rather a shortage – from all the farms and all the garland makers we had difficulty in putting together the thousand we sent you ... even picking the ones that should have been picked tomorrow. We had as many narcissi as you wanted so we sent you four thousand instead of two thousand you ordered.' The sheer amount of flowers ordered for the wedding ceremony itself is striking; we can only imagine how they could have arrived in a fresh state for the occasion.

At funerals the family of the deceased burnt incense for the time-honoured practical and religious reasons: dispelling the smell of death and honouring the gods. Incense was taken from the *acerra* or incense box and placed on the burning altar. The same word, *acerra*, is used to describe the miniature altar near the deceased on which incense was burned up until the day of burial. Garlands of flowers were placed around the body as it lay in state. Evidence for this practice is not only found in literary descriptions; funerary reliefs also bear testament to the importance of scent as part of the rites. Incense burners and garlands of fruit and flowers in abundance form part of the rich decoration on the Tomb of the Haterii, a family of builders who lived and worked in the second century AD. Lucian, a second-century AD satirist and rhetorician, recommends myrrh as a suitable scent at funerals. As part of the funeral service itself, small glass bottles or unguentaria (sometimes referred to as tear bottles in this context) were thrown on the funeral pyre. Misshapen by the heat of the fire, these small vessels are common finds among the detritus left behind by the Greeks and Romans. Finally, the ashes of the deceased were mixed with scented oils before being placed in an urn.

Prior to the adoption of Christianity, women were often buried with perfume vessels and other toilette accoutrements: mirrors, cosmetic pots and combs, for example. These were symbols of their daily life and routine. Other perfume vessels recovered from graves may have been used to dispense libations at the funeral itself. An elaborate perfume phial found in the grave of a young Roman lady buried in a lead coffin in Spitalfields in London is one such example. Given its shape and design it was probably used in the funeral ceremony and then buried with her thereafter. The vessel is certainly an ornate and expensive object, which in turn reflects the wealth and elevated social status of the occupant of the grave and her family.

Pliny the Elder deplores the excessive use of perfume at funerals. He lambasts Nero for having allegedly burned a whole year's worth of incense at the funeral of his wife Poppaea, who was not cremated but stuffed. In the words of the historian Tacitus (AD 56–c. 120), the empress was 'pickled [and] stuffed with perfumes after the custom of foreign rulers'. The historian's disdain is implicit. Poppaea died in AD 65, and both Pliny the Elder and Tacitus are her contemporaries, so it is tempting to think that they witnessed the funeral first hand. However, in the absence of proof we must temper such fancies with the acknowledgment that Poppaea generally receives a bad press from Roman authors.

## Perfume Pricing

> The iris is best in Elis, and at Cyzicus; the perfume made from roses is most excellent at Phaselis, and that made at Naples and Capua is also very fine. That made from crocuses is in the highest perfection at Soli in Cilicia, and at Rhodes. The essence of spikenard is best at Tarsus; and the extract of vine-leaves is made best in Cyprus and at Adramyttium. The best perfume from marjoram and from apples comes from Cos. Egypt bears the palm for its essence of Cyprus; and the next best is the Cyprian, and Phœnician, and after them comes the Sidonian.
>
> Apollonius of Herophila quoted in
> *Deipnosophistae*

There were scented waters, oils, powders and incense for sale all over the classical world. In many cases, the price of these goods was justifiably high. Popular contemporary methods of extraction (expression, maceration and enfleurage) did not provide a high yield. Certain plants were not geographically widespread and therefore needed to be imported, sometimes from far-off places. Inevitably, the cost of transport added to the cost of the goods at point of sale. For example, agarwood was purchased both from India and Arabia while balm of Gilead was imported from Judea. Some of the most expensive perfumes and ingredients to make perfume came from Arabia. Indeed, according to Pliny the Elder, 'Arabia is the sole producer of frankincense and even then not the whole of Arabia.' At the height of the Roman Empire, Alexandria in Egypt was an important centre of trade in luxury goods including perfume and especially frankincense. So precious was the resin that those working with it in the factories in Alexandria were routinely searched to make sure they were not absconding with any of it.

The Greeks and Romans did not always know the exact origin of the ingredients that they were so keen to obtain. Myths grew up around various perfume ingredients, and according to Pliny the Elder this inflated prices still further, as in the following example: 'In regard to cinnamon and cassia a fabulous story has been related by antiquity and first of all by Herodotus that they are obtained from birds nests and particularly that of the phoenix ... these tales having been invented by the natives to raise the price of these commodities.' The element of mystique that surrounded scent added not only to costs in the real world but also to increasing demand for an already expensive commodity.

There were other factors that affected the cost of perfumes. The Palmyrene Tariff is a record of the duties paid on goods entering and exiting the city of Palmyra, an important trading centre in Syria, from AD 137 during the reign of Emperor Hadrian. Written on huge stone tablets in both Greek and Aramaic, the tariff specified the taxes imposed on perfumes. It seems that different levels of tax could be charged on perfumes depending on how they were being transported to their destination; for instance, whether they were packed in alabaster containers or goatskin bags.

Inevitably, prices for scent did fluctuate and were subject to usual market forces of supply and demand. However, for some scents, such as spikenard and myrrh, the price might depend on the quality of the product. It is true to say that there were goods of inferior quality that were more affordable and allowed poorer people to imitate wealthier citizens. Pliny the Elder outlines the prices of the different grades of nard available from the most expensive to the cheapest:

Leaf nard varies in price according to the size; for that which is known by the name of hadrosphaerum consisting of larger leaves sells at 40 denarii per pound when the leaves are smaller it is called mesosphaerm and is sold at 60. but that which is considered the most valuable of all is known as microsphaerm and consists of the very smallest of leaves sells at 75 denarii per pound. All these varieties of nard have agreeable odour but it is most powerful when fresh.

These various grades of nard were used for softening as well as perfuming the skin, and we know that they were shipped in large, medium and small balls.

While specific perfumes fell in and out of fashion and prices went up and down to reflect this, some of the most desirable perfumes always fetched high prices. The market in luxurious products such as frankincense and cinnamon was brisk except in times of war or social upheaval, when the trade was curtailed. For example, during the Social Wars, fought between the Roman Republic and other cities and tribes in Italy from 91 BC to 87 BC, the sale of exotic unguents was actually forbidden.

## Homegrown Scent

> Still, the superior excellence of each perfume is owing to the purveyors and the materials and the artists and not to the place itself.
>
> Athenaeus of Naucratis, *Deipnosophistae*

Although many expensive scents came from beyond the Mediterranean, not all quality perfumes were imported. Homegrown products could also be of high quality and, as a result, very expensive. For example, perfume made of roses from the fertile region of Campania in south-western Italy, which includes the well-preserved towns Pompeii and Herculaneum, was considered superior to almost anything else. Indeed, in general terms, the area was highly regarded for the quality of its scent products. According to Pliny the Elder, 'in all other respects Egypt is of all the countries in the world best adapted for the production of unguents but Campania runs it close.'

Campania's soil was, and is, very fertile and there is clear evidence of mass production of perfumes there from the classical period. The discovery of many small glass perfume bottles in the grounds of a house in Pompeii, found alongside a number of larger jars or amphorae and a large terracotta funnel, suggests the presence of scent production on a commercial scale. Pollen analysis from this site, known as the Garden of Hercules (or, rather more prosaically, House II.viii.6), suggests that a variety of flowers including roses, violets and lilies were grown here. Frescoes from the House of the Vettii at Pompeii show cupids engaged in making perfume. Although the participants are mythological, the activity depicted likely reflects the daily business relating to this industry that went on in the town itself. The frescoes depict flatbed perfume presses, used to extract the fragrant oils, and physical examples of these presses have been found in the area too. In one of these frescoes a lady is depicted testing a perfume on her wrist. According to Theophrastus, 'perfumers as a rule apply their scents to customers' wrists', which he claims is done because perfumes are most pleasant when applied at that spot, perhaps because of the temperature of the skin. At a modern perfume counter people will often do the same.

## Perfume Traders

Solon (630 BC–*c.* 560 BC), an early and rather harsh Athenian statesman and lawmaker, passed a decree in 594 preventing men from trading in perfumes. He did so on the basis that scent was both overindulgent and effeminate. However, it would appear there was no penalty for contravening the legislation. In fact, the law was ignored because the financial gains to be made dealing in perfume were too great. Although, if we trust the words of Cicero, trade in general was never considered a respectable profession for members of elite society, that did not deter some members of the upper classes. There was money to be made in the trade of luxury goods whether homegrown or imported. Lucius Plautius Plancus (87 BC–15 BC), an ally of Julius Caesar (100 BC–44 BC), is one example of a member of the aristocracy being involved in the sale of scent. The Faenii, an elite family from Capua, also dealt in perfume: scent was one of the main industries of the town.

As the Roman Empire expanded, opportunities grew for the import of exotic flowers and herbs from beyond the boundaries of the empire. Arabian caravans provided a source – if not necessarily a regular one – of myrrh, frankincense and other exotic aromatics. Closer to home, at Pompeii, inscriptions bear witness to named perfumers who worked there. We know of an Agatho, a Phoebus and a Marcus Decidius Faustus. We know too of an Athenian perfumer named Peron and of course Cosmus, who crops up repeatedly in Martial's short poems. One Egyptian living in Athens owned three perfumery businesses. It was big business, and lucrative to boot.

## Shopping for Scent

Various sorts of shops stocked perfume, an indication of the variety of functions served by scent in the classical period. Among those who sold scent were druggists (*aromatarii* and *pharmacopalae*), incense peddlers (*thurarii*), and perfume and ointment makers (*unguentarii*). The *pigmentarius*, a merchant who dealt in pigments, dealt in perfumes too, as did barbershops. In Greece the word *myropolium* referred to the shop where fragrant ointments, balsams and essences were sold; the seller was known as the *myropola*. The word *myron* indicated a more expensive scent in Ancient Greece while *chrisma* was a cheaper product, perhaps a salve.

Shops that sold the same type of products were often grouped together in the same geographical area within a town or city. The shopping areas for perfume that we know of include the Seplasia, a street or square in the town of Capua in Campania. This area was renowned for its perfumed goods. Indeed, Seplasia and Seplasarius became names synonymous with perfume and perfumer sellers respectively. Capua was linked directly to Rome by the Appian Way, one of the main Roman thoroughfares. In the city of Rome itself, various streets specialised in certain goods. The Vicus Tuscus was later referred to as the Vicus Thurarius because of the number of perfume and incense sellers touting their wares there. The connecting street was known as the Vicus Unguentarius, literally 'street of perfumers'. In the Via Sacra, one of ancient Rome's other main thoroughfares, one could buy luxury goods including expensive perfumes, while the Subura in Rome, an area with a somewhat more bohemian but nevertheless fashionable reputation, housed a number of cosmetics and perfume shops.

The intense competition in the market for sale and purchase of scented oils and perfumes led some suppliers to engage in fraud. Pliny the Elder, commenting on the price of balsam, remarks, 'In no other case is more obvious fraud practised ... so much does it pay to increase the quantity by adulteration.' Expensive balsam was sometimes diluted with donkey milk. You could not always be sure what you were buying. Counterfeit goods were around then just as they are today.

## Mary Magdalene: Scent and Sainthood

> Then Mary took about a pint of pure nard. It was an expensive
> perfume. She poured it on Jesus' feet and wiped them with her hair.
> The house was filled with the sweet smell of the perfume.
>
> John 12:3

Scent features significantly in the New Testament and the life of Jesus, much as it had done in the books of the Old Testament, with the story of the washing of Jesus' feet perhaps the most well-known example. If nothing else, the tale certainly reinforces the monetary value of scent; the nard she applied was valued at 300 denarii, thought to be roughly the equivalent of a year's wages for a working man at this time.

Perfume is a key feature in the story of Mary Magdalene, who has sometimes been identified as the Mary in the account of the washing of the feet. She is often depicted holding a bottle or box of scent (*pyxis*) and is interpreted as symbolising both temptation and redemption. As one of the myrrh bearers (or *myrophorae*) she attends Christ's empty tomb. In the teachings of the Catholic Church, Mary Magdalene is the patron saint of contemplative life and of converts, glovers, hairdressers, penitent sinners, people ridiculed for their piety, perfumeries, pharmacists, tanners and women in general. Most of these guardianships have some connection with scent. Mary is believed to have received communion at the ancient Greek city of Ephesus on 22 July, the day recognised today as her feast day. She died at the altar immediately following that communion. According to tradition, the church smelled of perfume for seven days, signalling her arrival in heaven.

Other saints, like Mary, were marked out by fragrance or what became known as an aroma of sanctity. The reality may have been that the pleasant smells with which saints were associated came from the incense, unguents and perfumes that were used in funeral rites, which in turn were perhaps linked with descriptions of paradise as a scented garden. Pagan ideas did not just fade away but became mixed with Christian belief; scent was used to call upon saints to intercede on worshippers' behalf in the early church, following on from the use of incense in other established religions as a call to and a mark of the presence of the divine. The first Christian Roman emperor, Constantine (reigned AD 306–337), gave two gold incense burners and a stockpile of spices and aromatics to the basilicas of Saint Peter and Saint John the Lateran in Rome; perfume remained an essential part of religious worship thereafter.

## Some Classic(al) Scents

Some perfumes popular in the classical world are known to us by name from the works of Greek and Roman authors. For example, metopion was a strong scent made up of balanos oil and bitter almond and myrrh. Crocinon was based on saffron, the best coming from Aegina (one of the Saronic Greek islands) or

Cilicia (in southern Turkey). Megalium (in Greek megalaeion) was apparently named after its maker, a perfumer called Megallus. The main ingredients of this perfume were myrrh, cinnamon and cassia. Theophrastus, Pliny the Elder and Dioscurides all give recipes for megalium, but they are not identical. Dioscurides' version comprises balanos, burnt resin, myrrh oil, cinnamon and cassia, with alkanet added for colour. Theophrastus begged to differ, however:

> Megaleion, these authorities say, is compounded of burnt resin and oil of balanos, with which are mixed cassia cinnamon and myrrh. They add that this perfume and the Egyptian are the most troublesome to make, since no others involve the mixture of so many and such costly ingredients. To make megaleion, they say, the oil is boiled for ten days and nights, and not till then do they put in the resin and the other things, since the oil is more receptive when it has been thoroughly boiled.

Megalium was not only an expensive perfume but also a treatment for skin inflammation and battle wounds. Not everyone liked this strong scent, though; Theophrastus complained that sweet marjoram, spikenard and megaleion 'among costly perfumes' could cause headaches. He adds that 'most of the cheap ones have also this effect notably that one made from bay'. According to Athenaeus, 'the perfume called panathenaicum is made at Athens' and apparently was named for its place of production, but its ingredients are unclear. The aforementioned susinum remained a favourite as well. According to Pliny the Elder, susinum was 'made of lilies, oil of behen-nut, reed, honey, cinnamon, saffron and myrrh; and next is oil of cyprus, made of cyprus, omphacium, cardamom, reed, rosewood and southernwood; some people also add oil of cyprus and myrrh and all-heal; the best is that made at Sidon and the next best in Egypt. But if oil of sesame is added, the mixture will last as long as four years; and its scent is brought out by the addition of cinnamon.'

According to Pliny the Elder, top-quality cyprinum came from the banks of the River Nile and not from Cyprus as its name might suggest. This scent consisted of a mixture of henna, cardamom, cinnamon, myrrh and southernwood. Regalium, or royal perfume, contained around twenty ingredients including wild grape, spikenard, lotus, cinnamon, myrrh, gladiolus and marjoram – surely a heady and expensive mix fit for a king. This perfume was said to have been favoured by the kings of Parthia. Rhodium was a scent based on roses. The roses of Paestum in Campania (close to modern Naples) were particularly famous. Vrentheion, a concoction of musk and lavender, was imported from Turkey. Telinum was made of fresh olive oil, cyperus, calamus, yellow melilot, fenugreek, honey and sweet marjoram. It was the most fashionable perfume at the time of the comic poet Menander (342 BC–291 BC). A fragment of poetry that survives from two centuries later indicates that Julius Caesar favoured this perfume as well. Finally there is malabathrum, a cinnamon-like scent native to Egypt. Among other uses, according to Pliny, malabathrum 'is put under the tongue for sweetness of the breath, and it is put among cloths for it keeps them from moths and scents them sweetly'.

## Miscellaneous Recipes
### For a Rose Pomander Necklace

Pomanders of roses (which they call rhodides) are made in the following way. Take forty teaspoonfuls of fresh roses (which are beginning to fade) before they have absorbed any moisture, ten teaspoonfuls of Indian nard and six teaspoonfuls of myrrh. These are pounded into small pieces and made into little balls the size of half a teaspoonful, dried in the shade, and stored in a jar made without pitch, tightly corked all around. Some also add two teaspoons of costus and as much Illyrian iris, also mixing in Chian [from Scios in the Aegean Sea] wine with honey. This is used around women's necks instead of necklaces, dulling the unsavoury smell of sweat.

Dioscurides, *Materia Medica*

## For Megalium

[Megalium] was composed of oil of balanus, balsamum, calamus, sweet-rush, xylobalsamum, cassia, and resin. One peculiar property of this unguent is that it requires to be constantly stirred while boiling, until it has lost all smell: when it becomes cold, it recovers its odour.

Pliny the Elder, *Historia Naturalis*

# 4

# THE MEDIEVAL WORLD
## The Byzantines, the Art of Distillation and Scent in Arabic Medicine

*Of all the worldly goods three things are dearest to my heart;*
*perfume, women and prayer.*

Ibn Arabi (AD 1165–1240)

## Introduction

The medieval period or Middle Ages, as we refer to it, lasted from approximately the fifth century to the end of the fifteenth century. During this time, scent continued to play an important role in religious ceremony as well as serving as the basis of prophylactic medicine and potential cures for disease. Men and women, especially among the upper classes, carried on using perfume to keep themselves clean and to make themselves physically attractive. Fragrances were increasingly put to use as household cleaners and air fresheners at this time, as well as being used as flavourings in food. Perfumes largely remained expensive luxuries, so their use was confined for the most part to royal courts and the higher echelons of medieval society.

The Early Middle Ages (up until the ninth century) are sometimes viewed as a rather stagnant dismal era, a time of social and cultural decline, leading to the epithet of 'the Dark Ages'. As far as scent is concerned, early Christian doctrine saw luxurious and flamboyant lifestyles frowned upon and this had a deleterious effect on the personal use of fragrance. However, the story of perfume in this period is not without its high points. In the first place, medieval scientific experimentation brought about new developments in the manufacture of scent. Chief among these innovations was the perfection of the art of distillation. Although this process had been known as far back as the Bronze Age, it had never been widely used. Secondly, cultural exchange between east and west during the Muslim conquests following the death of prophet Mohammed in 632 and the Crusades from 1095 to 1492 facilitated knowledge of different perfumes and encouraged the use of a variety of ingredients across a wide geographical area. In truth, one cannot overplay the importance of smell in the Middle Ages.

There remained a genuine fear of bad odours at this time, borne in part from concern about disease. This anxiety was intensified further by the association of bad smells with Hell and damnation in the afterlife, a feature of both the Islamic and the Christian religions. In contrast to an eternal life of stinking misery in hell, Christians associated heaven with the sweet scent of flowers, grass and herbs, and in Islamic religion paradise was envisaged as a fragrant garden. On perhaps a lesser note, bad smells could even result in family break-up at the time. Hywel Dda, who ruled most of Wales from 942 to 948, decreed that bad breath was a legitimate reason for a wife to leave her husband. In short, as far as the people of the medieval period were concerned, a bad smell could have all sorts of unpleasant connotations and even profound consequences.

## Relevant Objects

The subject of scent crops up in a variety of medieval written sources including conduct manuals, medical texts, recipe books, household accounts and inventories, private letters and even legal documents. However, there is much less in the way of material evidence for perfume dating from this period, partly because

Christians were not routinely buried with grave goods. References to scent and perfume making can nonetheless be found in works of art, and some relevant artefacts have survived. For example, the Erfurt Treasure, a hoard found under an ancient wall in the town of Erfurt near Frankfurt in Germany, includes a silver perfume bottle dating from the fourteenth century. The cosmetic set of which this object is part probably belonged to a young Jewish woman of high status who would have worn it on the belt at her waist. Disappointingly, particularly as this is such a rare artefact, analysis of the bottle's contents has not been possible. Despite the best efforts of the L'Oréal Perfume Institute in Paris, there was just too little left in the bottle. However, it has been suggested that the bottle contained a mix of perfumed oil, perhaps rose or jasmine.

The San Marco incense burner is another perfume-related object dating from this period. Here we have an item of a deeply sacred nature. The burner may have arrived in Venice during the Fourth Crusade, perhaps around 1204. It is a highly decorative object; its stunning openwork design allowed the scented vapours burning within to escape and spread into the surrounding area. Finally, the eleventh-century Veroli Casket was probably crafted for a high-status individual at the Byzantine court at Constantinople. Made of wood and inlaid with ivory, the casket contains further boxes inside. One theory is that this luxurious container was used to store precious perfumes, though this is not certain.

## Perfume Preferences

Certain scents coveted in past centuries retained their prestige and value in the medieval period. Rose, lavender, iris, sweet flag, herbs like thyme and the dried peel of oranges and lemons were all popular. While cinnamon, costus, spikenard, frankincense and saffron maintained their share of the market, balsam and myrrh fell out of fashion. Camphor, ambergris and sandalwood imported from India were also valued for their fragrance. According to the ninth-century court physician Yuhanna ibn Masawaiyh, agarwood (or aloeswood as it is sometimes known) was one of the five most important fragrances alongside musk, camphor, ambergris and saffron. Derived from infected tree resin, agarwood was as prized in Arab culture then as it is today, while it is now known simply as oud. The resin features in both factual and fictional writings of the period, appearing as an ingredient in perfumes and as a standalone scent in contemporary medical recipes. It is also mentioned in *One Thousand and One Nights*: 'Her breath breathed ambergris and perfumery and her lips were sugar to taste and carnelian to see.'

Some fragrant plants assumed an emblematic importance, too. The lily and the rose were two of the most popular flowers in the Middle Ages. Both of these plants were imbued with symbolism, being closely associated with the Virgin Mary. The red rose symbolised her charity while both the rose and the lily represented her purity. Rosewater, rose petals and dried rosebuds were not only used for hand washing and freshening linen but were made into rosary beads as an aid to religious worship.

## The Byzantines

The Byzantine Empire comprised the remnants of the old eastern part of the Roman Empire and was centred on the city of Constantinople (modern Istanbul). The empire thrived from around AD 330 until its demise in AD 1453 when, just as had happened to the Roman Empire in the west, it too was overrun, in this case by the Ottomans. Constantinople itself was a hub for the import of the costliest perfumes and ingredients. The *Book of the Eparch*, sometimes referred to as the *Book of the Prefect*, is a particularly relevant source of information about the commercial life of the city. The Eparch was equivalent to the city mayor and the book itself is a collection of legal documents dating from the tenth century organising aspects of Byzantine economic life relating to the mercantile guilds. These medieval guilds were associations of craftsmen or merchants formed for commercial benefit.

The guilds could yield considerable economic and political power. In the tenth volume of the *Book of the Eparch* we find that the guild of the *myrepsoi* – dealers in drugs, perfumes and dyes – sold 'pepper, spikenard, cinnamon, aloe wood, ambergris, musk, frankincense, myrrh, balsam, indigo, lac, lapis lazuli, and yellow wood'. Clearly the members of the guild traded in quite a range of goods, many of them precious and expensive. Consequently, the quality of these products was strictly controlled at point of sale. Again, according to the *Book of the Eparch*:

> Every perfumer shall have his own shop, and not invade another's. Members of the guild are to keep watch on one another to prevent the sale of adulterated products. They are not to stock poor quality goods in their shops: a sweet smell and a bad smell do not go together. When the cargoes come in from Chaldaea [an area situated on the lower confluence of the rivers Tigris and Euphrates], Trebizond [the north eastern corner of Anatolia and Southern Crimea] or elsewhere, they shall buy from the importers on the days appointed by the regulations ... Importers shall not live in the City for more than three months; they shall sell their goods expeditiously and then return home.

In this same document we also find that from AD 895 perfumers had to use a small, very precise set of scales to weigh their expensive aromatics. Weighing scales and the accurate measurement of goods would have been important before this date, of course, but here we first find the use of accurate measures clearly enshrined in law. The *Book of the Eparch* also outlined the required siting of the perfumers' shops: 'Their stalls shall be placed in a row between the Milestone and the revered icon of Christ that stands above the Bronze Arcade, so that the aroma may waft upwards to the icon and at the same time fill the vestibule of the Royal Palace.' Clearly the smell emanating from these premises continued to fulfil the long-held dual purposes of honouring both divine and earthly rulers.

## Scent at the Byzantine Court

The Byzantine rulers, both male and female, were known for their personal love of perfume. In the early seventh century, Jabala VI, ruler of the Ghassanids, a Byzantine client state in the Levant, is described by a visitor to his court as sitting 'upon a spread for drinking under it were myrtle and jasmine and other sorts of aromatics and he was daubed with ambergris and musk'. In the tenth century it is known that aloe, musk, amber and frankincense were among the Byzantine emperor's baggage on military expeditions and that perfume was a feature of imperial processions through the city of Constantinople at this time. Constantine Porphyrogenitus, Byzantine emperor from 913 to 959, used rosewater to scent all the rooms in his palace.

The Byzantine emperors not only used perfume on their person and property but also bestowed it upon on others too. Guests arriving at court would have their rooms heavily scented and bowls of rosewater provided for their use. Two apples tied fastened to cinnamon sticks formed a traditional gift from the emperor to persons deemed worthy of his attentions. An eleventh-century text entitled *Book of Treasures and Gifts* records the courtly and diplomatic exchanges of presents including musk, aloe and camphor. The gift of perfume from the rulers of Byzantium to other leaders and vice versa was common practice. In 1188, Sultan Saladin even sent Byzantine Emperor Isaac II (reigned 1185–1195) one hundred musk sacs and a live musk deer. In a religious context, perfume and scented textiles were particularly coveted offerings.

## The Empress Zoe

Her own private bedroom was no more impressive than the workshops in the market where the artisans and the blacksmiths toil, for all round the room were burning braziers, a host of them.

Each of her servants had a particular task to perform: one was
allotted the duty of bottling the perfumes, another of mixing them,
while a third had some other task of the same kind.

Michael Psellos (*c.* 1017–1078)

Empress Zoe Porphyrogenita (meaning 'born into the purple',
of royal birth) ruled the Byzantine Empire from 1028 until her
death in 1050. Like other members of elite Byzantine society,
she certainly valued scent. However, Zoe took that interest a
step further, actively engaging in the perfume-making process.
In the words of monk, philosopher, politician and historian
Michael Psellos, 'her one and only concern at this time, the
thing on which she spent all her energy, was the development of
new species of perfumes, or the preparation of unguents. Some
she would invent, others she improved.' Zoe, together with her
younger sister Theodora, converted part of the imperial palace
at Constantinople into a perfume workshop or *myrepseion*. Here
they conducted their own experiments. In order to create her
perfumes, Zoe imported exotic ingredients from India and Egypt
including frankincense, musk, cedarwood and camphor. In fact,
what she was doing was dabbling in alchemy, the precursor of
modern chemistry.

Some thought that the empress concocted poisons in her
rooms alongside legitimate perfumes; certainly at least one of
her husbands died in mysterious circumstances. It is true that
medieval historians are wont to make reference to the empress's
fascination with luxury perfumes (and possible poisons) to tarnish
her reputation. However, according to Psellos, Zoe's fascination
with herbs and spices may not have been so much in the pursuit
of luxury but instead pertaining to her religious beliefs. In his
words, 'One thing above all claimed her attentions and on this
she expended all her enthusiasm – the offering of sacrifices to
God. I am not referring so much to the sacrifice of praise, or of
thanksgiving, or of penitence, but to the offering of spices and
sweet herbs, the products of India and Egypt.'

## *Arabic Medicine*

> Prescription of medicine to cut sweat: the body is cleaned with rose
> fat and butchers broom fat, then rosewater is poured on it and then
> it is fanned.
>
> Ibn al-Tilmidh (1074–1165)

Arabic medical treatments of the time predominantly relied on aromatic plants and herbs, and it is true to say that much of what earlier civilisations had previously understood about the making of scent and its use, no doubt in view of the already long-established association between perfume and medicine, was preserved in contemporary Arabic medical texts. As unpleasant odours continued to be interpreted as a sign of disease, either masking or counteracting a bad smell with a pleasant scent was a first line of defence. Indeed, the power of aromatics remained the only means of defence against disease and ill health in a world without antibiotics and the benefits of modern medical science.

Doctors used pungent herbs, fragrant flowers and sweet-smelling resins in a number of ways and for a number of different illnesses. Headaches could be treated with the scent of roses, lavender, sage or hay, for example. Aromatics were prescribed to relieve the pain of arthritis, and resins such as frankincense and myrrh might be applied to sores. Lavender was used to scent bedclothes as an aid to sleep; this is, of course, still a popular remedy for insomnia today. The early Byzantine physician Alexander of Tralles (525–605) prescribed aromatic pastilles for a fever, while the Persian physician Mesue (*c.* 777–857) even used incense as an anaesthetic – a nod perhaps to the potential of burning resins, such as frankincense, to calm the mind. The Persian physician and alchemist Al Razi (854–925) recommended the following as an effective deodorant for a man: 'One should coat his body with leaves of Cypress-tree and the oil of its flowers.' The seventh-century Byzantine physician Paulus of Aegina (*c.* 625–690), who wrote a seven-volume medical encyclopaedia, recommended fragrance for just about everything from healing wounds to treating cancer.

Nicholas Myrepsos, who is believed to have been the physician to thirteenth-century Byzantine emperor John Vatrazis, wrote a work entitled *Dynameron* which included some 2,000 recipes, among them formulas for making perfume for medicinal purposes. Some of these recipes were preserved from earlier books that are now lost, while some can be attributed to Nicholas himself. Even his name suggests that perfumes were his speciality: *Myrepsos* in ancient Greek literally means 'preparer of unguents'. His work includes recipes for oil of nard as a perfume and incense, which he also prescribed as a sedative.

According to the Muslim Polymath Avicenna (980–1037), a pleasant smell was even considered proper etiquette for those who practised medicine: 'The doctor should make the patient happy, amusing him, and sitting in places with moderate climate, moisten the air of his house and perfume it with sweet fragrance; in general he should always smell sweet odours.'

## Scent and Islam

The taking of a bath on Friday is compulsory for every male Muslim who has attained the age of puberty and also the cleaning of his teeth and the using of perfume if it is available.

Hadith 879

Trade with the east brought new methods of production as well as new ingredients into the west. However, many ancient traditions pertaining to scent were maintained as part of Islamic culture too. Just like the Ancient Egyptian temples, mosques were built with a fragrance (musk, for example) embedded in the mortar. Perfume was sprinkled at public gatherings and used on a more personal level to anoint the hair and beard. In Islamic tradition, women wore perfume within their domestic confines but were forbidden from attracting the attention of others by giving off a strong fragrance and tempting men other than their husbands when outside the home. Feminine fragrances considered appropriate for use by Muslim women included scents based on saffron, turmeric and myrtle. On the other hand, camphor was deemed suitable for men while yellow saffron was discouraged for them. Olive oil and sesame oil were applied to hair, while the stronger-scented ben oil and violet were applied to the body. The conurbations of Damascus, Shiraz and Jur were all famous for perfume production under the Abbasids. Perfume was still regarded as prestigious, and some scents were reserved for the social elite. The ninth-century caliph Al Mutawakkil (ruled 847–861) thought the rose was the king of sweet-scented flowers and that only those of his exalted rank were worthy of it.

## Abulcasis, Al-Kindi and the Art of Distillation

We know that ancient civilisations were familiar with distilling, a method of separating liquid from solid by heating to bring about evaporation and condensation. While this was recognised as a way of producing alcohol, it was also the means by which fragrant oils could be extracted from even the most delicate of plants. Attar (or Otto) is the transliteration of the Arabic word *itr*, used to refer to the fragrant oil that can be extracted from flowers using this method. King Zimri-Lim, who ruled the Mesopotamian city of Mari from about 1775 to 1761 BC, used distillation to make perfumes and incense from cedar, cypress, ginger and myrrh. However, despite awareness of this technique at this very early date, the process had not been widely practised until Avicenna developed steam distillation. Later, around 1320, the serpentine cooler was invented in Italy and further improved the process.

Although it typically took a lot of raw ingredients to make a small amount of scent – a fact that contributed to many perfumes remaining a luxury – the process of distillation allowed for the production of even the more subtle of scents in larger quantities, marking a milestone in the history of perfume production. Greater use could be made of certain fragile scents and aromatics such as jasmine and sandalwood. The process of distillation perfected the production of rosewater in particular; the scent of roses was already much beloved by the Arabs, and it would be appreciated by many others in the centuries to come.

In his writings, Abulcasis (AD 936–1013), a physician, surgeon and chemist living and working in the Spanish city of Cordoba, not only gives us detailed descriptions of the equipment used in the process of distillation but devotes an entire book (his nineteenth treatise) to the subject of perfumes. He records expensive perfumes meant for the caliph and the wealthy elite as well as moderate and even cheap varieties. His recipes include both simple and compound mixtures, and he details more than a hundred perfumes, giving each a variety of uses including fresheners for clothes, vapour rubs for respiration and slow-burning incense for fumigation. Abulcasis even specifies the perfumes suited to different seasons of the year: those based on camphor or rose he considered best for summer, while musk preparations were better suited to the winter months. He also classified different smells in a way similar to that employed by modern perfumers.

The philosopher, mathematician and physician Al-Kindi (AD 801–873) wrote extensively about fragrant essential oils too. His *Book of Perfume, Chemistry and Distillation* contains over one hundred recipes for scented waters, aromatic oils and salves made from flowers such as hyacinth and rose as well as fruits like apricot and apple. He includes recipes that use animal excretions too, most notably ambergris and musk. In his description of equipment needed to make a perfume Al-Kindi gives pride of place to the alembic. The word *alembic* in Arabic literally means 'cup beaker'. It is, in fact, a dual vessel with a connecting tube. Invented by Jabir ibn Hayyan (AD 721–813), who incidentally earned himself the title of the Father of Chemistry, Hayyan's alembic along with his experiments concerning evaporation, filtration and distillation were central to the development of the perfume industry. He also wrote two treatises on the subject.

By 1100, alcohol was being distilled in the west (at Salerno in Italy, for example) and used primarily as a base for perfumes and medicines.

## The Trade in Aromatics

For centuries, Arab traders travelling along the Silk Road had sold their exotic spices, expensive resins, fragrant woods and aromatic herbs to the west. These were the middlemen when it came to selling perfume and perfume ingredients from the east, in particular India and China, to countries in eastern Europe. By the ninth century, perfumes and their necessary ingredients also entered Europe by sea along the incense and spice routes which connected the Mediterranean with countries to the east and to the south. Luxury goods were shipped from Byzantium to Venice and via Baghdad to Spain. Venice in particular became an important trading hub; given its geographical position the city became, quite literally, the economic gateway into Europe. Musk, ambergris, cloves, camphor, sandalwood and aloeswood were traded extensively for use in fragrance at this time.

Popular scents like eau de Chypre (dating from 1191), a flower water made from a mixture of gums, resins and spices including labdanum, storax and calamus with a rosewater base, was brought to Europe by the returning crusaders. When Richard the Lionheart, who ruled in England from 1189 to 1199, returned to England from Cyprus in 1194 he brought various gums, resins and rosewater with him.

Family alliances in the form of marriage links helped to spread the popularity of scent too. The marriage of Princess Theodora Doukaina, daughter of Byzantine emperor Constantine X Dukas, to Domenico Selvo, the Doge of Venice, took place in 1060. The marriage not only helped promote east–west trade links but advanced the burgeoning interest in perfumery at the Venetian court itself. The Venetian explorer and adventurer Marco Polo (1254–1324) would be instrumental in bringing musk, a scent much favoured by the Arabs, to the west. It could be traded either in its original state (the animal's sac) or decanted into another flask or container. Transport costs still represented a considerable hurdle, and it would be the very end of the medieval period before musk became as popular in the west as it was in the east. In his book about his travels, *Il Milone*, Marco Polo also remarked upon ambergris, 'voided from the entrails of whales', as merchandise in high demand. Perfume remained a much coveted and expensive commodity.

## Christianity and Holy Incense

> We offer incense to you Christ God as a sweet fragrance. Having received it on your super celestial altar send down upon us in return the grace of your all holy spirit.
>
> Symeon of Thessalonica (1381–1429)

Because of the strong link between fragrance and the old pantheistic religions, the Christian church showed some reluctance at first in adopting scent as part of its worship. That is to say, as incense had been very much part of what was now deemed heathenism, its use in a Christian setting was thought to send the wrong message. The early Christian church even warned against excessive use of perfumes on the grounds that these had the potential to corrupt the soul. There were those in the early church who feared that indulging the senses would lead to being corrupted by the sins of the world, and some took this belief to the extreme. These ascetics, as they were known, exercised strict control over their own bodies, rejecting cleanliness and pleasant smells. However, even by the beginning of the Middle Ages the church had overcome much of its fear in respect of the use of scent, and the burning of incense as part of Christian ritual quickly embedded itself. As early as Constantine's rule in the fourth century there was a budget set aside for the regular use of spikenard and balsam in churches, with further funding reserved for spices and incenses on special holy days.

Perfume thus became an important part of religious worship once more, fulfilling the need to both honour God and establish a relationship with him. Sweet fragrances suggested the actual presence of God in the church, very much in the tradition of the pantheistic religions of Ancient Egypt and the other Bronze Age civilisations. Ironically, despite the initial reservations about perfume in some quarters, the Christian church as a whole would do much to preserve its use in the west. Not only incense but the holy oil used to anoint in church ceremony was often perfumed. Lamps in churches contained oil scented with nard or rose. Abbey gardens bloomed with scented flowers and herbs including lavender, rosemary and sage. In Christian belief, as in earlier religions, smell formed an integral part of the medieval interpretation of heaven and hell, and by making use of incense and scented anointing oil the church was attempting to recreate paradise on earth.

One of the main dispensers of scent in a medieval church setting was the swinging censer or thurible. This was – and, in Roman Catholic and Orthodox denominations, remains – central to worship. The thurible is a container suspended on chains made of precious metal and decorated with religious imagery. Inside, incense burns on embers and the perfumed smoke escapes through the holes in the vessel to fill the surrounding area. In the Middle Ages these thuribles wafted their contents, in particular frankincense and myrrh, across the assembled congregation. Both the swinging motion and the fumes of the burning resins helped to create a sense of religious fervour. In the thirteenth century an exceptionally large and magnificent thurible was installed in the Santiago de Compostela Cathedral in Galicia, Spain. This particular site marked the end of the route taken by pilgrims known as the Camino de Santiago (the Way of St James). The route led to the remains of St James the Great, believed to be housed within the cathedral itself. It is easy to see how the smell of incense at the end of the journey might have soothed and revived the pilgrims.

The profusion of perfume might also have disguised the odour of so many unwashed bodies after their arduous trek.

## Saints and the Odour of Sanctity

Aside from representing godliness and heaven on earth, fragrance was also, on occasion, given to worshippers on holy days and feast days as miracle cures. That is to say, fragrant oil poured on relics was often saved and dispensed to pilgrims (for a charge) as a cure-all which they could take home. Scent was a crucial element of its healing power. No doubt this was a distinctly lucrative business enterprise as far the church was concerned. A saint whose corpse was believed to exude scent that could heal was termed a myroblyte. One example is Saint Demetrius, who was martyred in the early fourth century AD and whose tomb began to pour forth perfume in the tenth century following the destruction of the church containing his relics in the Aegean port city of Thessaloniki.

That a pleasant smell could be a test of sanctity was an idea inherited from antiquity. Saints, just like their predecessors, the gods and goddesses of the classical world and divinities honoured by Bronze Age religions, not only welcomed scent as part of worship but exuded sweet perfume themselves and even fed on fragrance for sustenance. The collecting or acquiring of religious relics became a bit of a craze in the medieval period. In order to decide whether a given piece of a saint's body, a piece of the true cross or whatever form the relic might take was in fact genuine, scent was used as a test of authenticity – the so-called odour of sanctity again.

Anecdotal accounts of the theft of relics mention that it was, on occasion, the sweet smell of perfume that raised the alarm as soon as the relic was disturbed. The story goes that this was what happened when a group of merchants tried to steal the remains of St Nicholas from his tomb in the town of Myra (now called Demre) in Turkey in the year 1087. The smell alerted the townsfolk to the theft as it was in progress.

There may, in fact, be some quite understandable and practical reasons why bones and other sanctified objects radiated a fragrant odour. In the first place, relics were often kept close to the altar in an area where incense was stored or used. Secondly, there were occasions when the relic or relics themselves might be anointed with holy oil which was of course scented. For both these reasons it is not surprising that relics smelled fragrant.

Very important secular and religious members of medieval society, revered churchmen and members of royalty or the aristocracy for example, might have their bodies embalmed with sweet-smelling spices so that the body could lie in state for some days without offensive odour. As the body was not always buried in one piece, nor indeed necessarily all in the same place, a single part might be preserved in this way too. The Scottish poet John Barbour (1320–1395) in his narrative poem *The Bruce* makes this claim with regard to Robert the Bruce, King of the Scots: 'His heart was removed from his body and embalmed, that is prepared with spices and perfumes, that it might remain long fresh and uncorrupted.'

## Rosary Beads and Scented Candles

The profusion of perfume in a church setting came not only from the burning of incense or indeed from the fragrant bones of saints but also from the scented candles that burned and the rosary beads worked in the hands of the worshippers. Gregory of Tours (AD 538–594), historian and bishop, wrote that in Reims on the occasion of the baptism of Clovis, King of the Franks, 'sticks of incense gave off clouds of perfume. Sweet-smelling candles gleamed bright and the holy place of baptism was filled with divine fragrance.' The scene he evokes is one of wonder that appeals to all the senses and in particular, I think, that of smell. Even when death was unexpected or there was some reason for haste, fragrance was a must. The death of Thomas a Becket, Archbishop of Canterbury, who was murdered in 1170, was certainly sudden and his burial took place without time to embalm his body, but tradition recounts that the church was filled with perfume nonetheless.

## The Monastery Garden

> Amongst my herbs sage holds the place of honour; of good scent it
> is full of virtue for many ills.
>
> Walafrid Strabo (*c.* AD 808–849)

Christian monastic religious orders divided their cloister grounds into physic and kitchen gardens. Flowers and herbs were grown in physic gardens as medicines and in kitchen gardens as foods, though flowers in particular might also be grown simply for their beauty. The monks themselves were well versed in medical treatments and the monastery was one port of call for anyone who was sick and in need of medical attention. The fragrance of the plants they grew was an essential part of their value in healing sickness and treating disease. Benedictine monk Walafrid Strabo had a particular favourite: 'Far and away the best of all in power and fragrance ... no man can remember how many uses there are for oil of roses as a cure for mankind's ailments.' High praise indeed, but the rose was just one plant with healing qualities associated with its smell. There were many others. Popular fragrant herbs grown to treat diseases included sage, anise, coriander, flax, mugwort, rue and yarrow.

## Soap and Sweet Waters

In the medieval period, soap was a pretty basic commodity made of wood ashes and tallow or animal fat. It was a caustic substance more often used to wash clothes than to clean one's body, with a rather unappealing black colour and a very strong odour. However, by 1200 there was Castile soap, made with olive oil and pot ash (not to be confused with potash) and imported from Spain. Popular across Europe, it was a luxury item much sought after by those who could afford it. Fragrant oils such as oil of lavender were added to the fat and pot ash to make this luxury soap appealing. Soap making is known in Britain from the eleventh century, and by the thirteenth century the industry was flourishing in large towns and cities, particularly Bristol, Coventry and London.

A mixture of hyssop (an aromatic herb of the mint family) and bay leaves was used as a deodorant. However, a sweet water was another way of keeping oneself smelling clean. Fruit- and flower-based waters such as rosewater, orange water, lemon water and jasmine water were very popular. Sweet waters were used especially to wash one's hands before, during and after meals. The elite members of Byzantine society ate with forks, but in the west this was considered effete so rich and poor alike ate with their hands. Clearly it made sense to keep one's hands as clean as possible. One household book that survives from the Middle Ages, entitled *Le Ménagier de Paris* (The Good Man of Paris), gives us some details. The text, penned around 1393 by a rather elderly gentleman as an instruction manual for his very young wife, suggests washing one's hands at the dinner table with water fragranced with herbs such as chamomile, marjoram, rosemary or sage. The old gentleman, who identifies himself only as 'a citizen of Paris', writes, 'Set sage to boil then pour out the water and let it cool until it is just warm. or you may instead use chamomile or marjoram or you may put in rosemary and boil them with orange peel. And bay leaves too are good.' Presumably the choice of herb would depend on seasonal availability as well as personal preference.

## Bathing

Although the practice of talking a bath was neither universal nor a regular undertaking in western Europe in the Middle Ages, it was by no means unknown. Indeed, bathing was considered a potential cure for disease. Hot steam baths or vapour baths (a hot water tub with aromatic herbs added) were used to literally 'smoke' the sick in order to cure them of their illness. Vapour and herb baths as a medical treatment are recorded in the Saxon text *Bald's Leechbook*, the oldest surviving English herbal, which dates from between AD 900 and 950. This book, which was probably the personal manual of a Saxon doctor, includes among other things instructions for preparing a herbal bath as a cure for blotch, thought to be some sort of skin disease:

> Boil the herbs ten times and separately in a basin: betony, lesser calamint, white horehound, agrimony, yarrow, mint, elecampane, hemp agrimony, knapweed, common centaury, dill, wild celery, fennel, equal amounts of each, then make a stool of three woods perforated underneath (the seat), sit over a basin, and blanket yourself over with a garment in case the steam escapes, pour [the decoction] into the basin under the stool, you might use those herbs three times, and stir underneath with a stick if you want it hotter, and before the bath smear the body and the face with sweet water and scramble two eggs in hot water, smear all the body with that.

The German abbess, mystic and composer Hildegard of Bingen (1098–1179) was even more specific as to the benefits of fragrant steam baths in her advice, holding that 'aromatic vapour baths are useful in the treatment of female disorders.' Avicenna also prescribed hot baths for particular complaints, recommending a bath fragranced with dill to cure intestinal problems and with bay leaves to treat urinary complaints.

Aside from its medicinal benefits, bathing in scented waters could also be a sexually stimulating experience. The *Decameron*, penned by the Italian author Giovanni Boccaccio (1313–1375), is a collection of one hundred tales about the nature of man at the time of the Black Death. It contains the following elaborate and sensual description of bathing:

> The lady herself washed Salabaetto all over with soap scented with musk and cloves. She then had herself washed and rubbed down by the salves. This done the slaves brought two fine and

very white sheets so scented with roses that they seemed like roses the slaves wrapped Salabaetto in one and the lady in the other and then carried them both on their shoulders to the bed ... They then took from the basket silver vases of great beauty some of which were filled with rose water some with orange water some with jasmine water and some with lemon water which they sprinkled on them.

Sex is very much a theme of the *Decameron* as a whole, and the luxurious and sensuous nature of this scene is greatly enhanced by the intoxicating range of fragrances mentioned.

## The Smell of the Plague: The Black Death

> ... and so many died that all believed that it was the end of
> the world.
> Agnolo di Tura del Grasso, *The Plague in Siena:*
> *An Italian Chronicle* (1348)

It is clear that the people of the Middle Ages were not the great unwashed that we once thought. Instead, they strove to keep themselves and their towns and cities free from disease without the help of modern medicine and with a limited understanding of how disease spread. Therefore, when the Black Death, also known as the Great Plague, arrived in Europe in 1347 it was not long before it took hold. Among the measures taken to prevent its spread, the English monarch Edward III (1312–1377) ordered the Mayor of London to rid the city of bad smells as noxious odours were believed to contribute to the spread of the plague. Saltpetre and brimstone were burnt to counteract it.

Other, somewhat more pleasant scents were also put to work. The fourteenth-century physician John of Burgundy recommended smelling 'roses, violets [or] lilies as both a protection against and a cure for the plague'. Boccaccio remarked that 'some people walked everywhere with fragrances and nose-coverings'. Women in particular carried small bunches of flowers or nosegays and other scented objects to ward off the foul pestilence. A nosegay consisted of a tightly tied small bunch of flowers, quite likely the very roses, violets and lilies recommended by John of Burgundy. These were held close to the nose to ward off the bad air believed to carry the disease. This practice survived on into Tudor times, and today the word is still used in connection with wedding flowers.

## Plague Waters

Plague water was the name given to various scented medicinal waters that were believed to be effective against the ravages of the disease. These probably came into being around 1370. Hungary water was one of the first. Possibly named after a queen consort of Hungary, Elisabeth of Poland (1305–1380), its original purpose is said to have been to preserve this lady's youthful appearance. Tradition has it that the treatment was so effective that young men sought the queen's hand in marriage even when she was aged seventy.

Aside from its reputation as an elixir of youth, Hungary water quickly became established as a notable protection against the plague too. The water could be consumed internally, used to wash oneself or worn as a perfume. It was, in fact, the first alcohol-based perfume and bears a greater similarity to our modern fragrances than the scented oils, aromatics and greasy solid or semi-solid mixtures that had gone before. The original form is thought to have consisted of rosemary, rosewater, orange flower water, verbena and mint. The best-quality Hungary water needed to be aged for six months, which was surely a disadvantage if you were seeking instant help in warding off the plague. Although Hungary water remains the best known, however, it was not the only plague water on the market. Other medicinal scented waters included Eau de Carmes (water of the Carmelites). This was a mixture of herbal oils including angelica and melissa, made from around 1379 at the Abbey of St Juste in France.

## Scenting the Home

> For me at the start of summer you put forth the beauty of
> your purple flower [the purple iris] ... With your help too the
> laundryman can stiffen his shining linen and scent it sweetly.
> Walafrid Strabo, *Hortulus*

For those who could afford them, flowers and strong-smelling herbs were used widely in domestic settings not only to rid the air of bad odours and ward off disease but also to protect clothing from destructive insects, to enhance the taste of food and to wash clothes. In the houses of the wealthy there were bowls of rosewater on tables for washing hands not only for hygiene purposes but also to rid one's hands of the pungent smell and grease of some of the strong-smelling food that was on the menu at this time. *Bald's Leechbook* recommended that scented garlands should be worn and displayed in the home. Bowls of potpourri consisting of iris mixed with orange and lemon peel were placed in rooms to freshen the air. As ever, bedclothes were infused with lavender to promote a good night's sleep. Fragrances could be multifunctional in a domestic context; the seventh-century physician Paulus of Aegina describes infusions of lilies in wine known as *oenantharia* (a product that took forty days to prepare), noting, 'The *oenantharia* are used by some solely for their fragrance and for luxury alone these persons having them poured over their bodies after coming out of the bath and having their tables wiped with sponges dipped in them.'

Rose petals in cloth bags kept clothes fragrant when in storage, while wormwood and rosemary acted as moth repellents. Strong-smelling rue might be put among clothing and linens to deter insects too. Violets or iris root gave clothes a pleasant fragrance. According to *The Good Man of Paris*, 'Roses of Provence are the best for putting in dresses but you should dry them in mid-August sift them so that the worms fall through the holes in the sieve. Then scatter them on the dresses.' The author's instructions are precise. Iris root had the added benefit of stiffening linen, as Walafrid points out in the quote above. The long mantles worn by well-to-do women in the Middle Ages might even have been lined with scented fur.

The household accounts of English ruler Edward IV (1442–1483) include sweet flowers, herbs and roots to be placed among the king's robes 'to make them breathe most wholesomely and delectable'. In Edinburgh Castle, prior to the fifteenth century, the so-called clerk of the wardrobe was responsible for the safe keeping of the king's valuables in his chamber. These valuables included perfumes and aromatics. In the grander medieval houses there were quarters known as still rooms or distillery rooms for preparing not only wine and beer but also medicines and scented waters. The still room was usually the responsibility of the lady of the household in the medieval period.

## Fragrant Food and Drink

The aromatics prescribed as treatments for various illnesses also served to counteract bad breath, for which *Bald's Leechbook* recommends aromatic drinks and fragrant mouthwashes. However, scented drinks had other medicinal benefits too. An anonymous Andalusian cookbook dating from the thirteenth century describes a drink made from syrup of fresh roses, a mixture of roses boiled in water 'for a day and a night' and then cooled and mixed with sugar. 'Cook all this until it takes the form of syrup. Drink one part syrup to two parts hot water ... its benefits are at the onset of dropsy and it fortifies the stomach and the liver and other internal organs and lightens the constitution; in this it is admirable.'

The same cookbook also suggests that 'whoever cooks lavender with wine, or if the person has no wine, with honey and water, and drinks it often lukewarm, it will alleviate the pain in the liver and in the lungs and the steam in his chest. Lavender wine will provide the person with pure knowledge and a clear understanding.' Such benefits were not to be scoffed at when little else of any potency was available.

Scent might be added to drinks simply to improve the taste, though fragrance sometimes acted as a preservative too. The Greeks and Romans had perfumed their wine in order to add to the flavour and to help preserve its quality – myrrh being a popular choice – and possibly in order to avoid the effects of drinking too much. In the medieval period wine might be spiced with marjoram. Alcoholic drinks were not the only ones to be spiced up. The newly discovered drink of coffee was laced with cardamom. When it comes to food, we find that rose petals were an ingredient in rose honey, rose syrup and rose sugar. The honey and sugar were prepared simply by mixing in rose petals and leaving them to infuse. Also, lavender and orange flower water were popular ingredients in the puddings served at the dinner tables of the well-to-do.

## Scenting the Floors

Medieval floors were carpeted with rushes and straw, if they were covered at all. Although this added warmth to a room and soaked up any moisture, the rushes and straw were not necessarily changed regularly and so could harbour bugs and mites. In order to repel these insects and, in so doing, limit the spread of disease and create a nicer living space, fragrant herbs were mixed with the aforesaid rushes and straw. As people walked across the floor these scented plants exuded a pleasant odour which acted as a counter to any nasty smells. Fennel, rosemary and sweet woodruff were among the herbs and flowers found in better-class private homes and public buildings. Scattering southernwood on floors was also considered an effective way of masking bad smells.

On special occasions flowers and aromatic herbs were thrown before important visitors as they processed; perhaps lavender, roses, violets or sweet flag. In England it was the job of the Royal Herb Strewer to ensure that noxious smells were kept away from the king and his entourage. The floors at the court of King Stephen (1096–1154) were regularly spread with rushes and flowers so that his knights need not sit on bare flagstones. Thomas à Becket too gave instructions that his hall floors should be covered each day with May blossom in spring and sweet-scented rushes in summer.

## Portable Perfume

The pomander, a scented ball of fat, became popular during the medieval period and endured for at least two centuries. The fad is said to have begun when in 1174 King Baldwin IV of Jerusalem (1161–1185) presented the Holy Roman Emperor Fredrick Barbarossa (1122–1190) with a pomander, which was until then unknown in the west. The ball of fat was typically scented with aromatic herbs and animal excretions such as musk, civet or ambergris, and its name comes from the French *pomme d'ambre* (literally 'apple of amber'), reminding us perhaps of the small balls of amber that aristocratic Roman ladies held in their hands and rubbed to give off a pleasing scent. In the medieval period the chief function of the pomanders was to ward off disease; at the height of its popularity the pomander even topped the traditional cane carried by physicians. Pomanders were also believed to protect against witchcraft and from the thirteenth century onward were considered acceptable as diplomatic gifts and tribute payments. Tied around the neck or attached to a belt, jewel-encrusted gold or silver pomanders quickly became a symbol of wealth and status.

Wealthy medieval citizens prized scented jewellery for its aesthetic appeal. Rosaries, the strings of beads on which Catholic prayers are counted, were originally made of dried rosebuds or resin beads. Necklaces, brooches and the like might have had little compartments hidden within them where a scent, perhaps a piece of cloth imbued with perfume, could be kept. Inhaling the fragrance emanating from these items of jewellery was believed to enhance one's mood as well as warding off disease and evil spirits.

## Perfume: Poison and Protection against Evil

Bad smells remained associated with evil, and perfumes were still used in magic to ward off evil beings in all their forms, as evident in the following recipe from the medieval period:

> Make a salve against the elfin race and against nocturnal demons and against the women whom the fiend cohabits with. Take the female hop-plant, wormwood, bishopswort, lupine, vervain, henbane, hare wort [hartwort], viper's bugloss, whortleberry plants, crow-leek [unidentified], garlic, hairif grains, [unknown] cockle, and fennel. Put the herbs into a vessel, place them under the altar, sing nine masses over them, boil them in butter and in sheep's grease, add plenty of consecrated salt, strain through a cloth; throw the herbs into running water. If any wicked temptation come to a man, or an elf or a nocturnal demon [assail him], smear his forehead with this salve, and put some on his eyes and some where his body is sore; and perfume him with incense, and repeatedly sign him with the sign of the cross.

This is fanciful stuff to many today, but it would not have seemed so in a time when pagan traditions existed alongside the established Christian religion.

Our aforementioned Byzantine princess, Zoe, was not the only famous lady accused of using perfume as a cover for poison. Eleanor of Aquitaine (1122–1204), the queen consort of France and subsequently England, favoured violets but was rumoured to have murdered Rosamund Clifford, the king's mistress, with poison concealed in attar of roses. Elsewhere, the fruit and seeds of cardamom, the scent of which was believed to be a powerful aphrodisiac, were used as love potion known as the Fire of Venus.

## Perfume and Theatre

It is in the medieval period that perfume begins to appear frequently in plays and literature, whether as a prop or as a major plot device. Some dramas even contained scenes devoted to the subject of scent.

The Digby Mary Magdalene, first performed sometime between 1480 and 1530, is a biography of the eponymous Mary who is herself closely associated with perfume and cosmetics. Mary the mother of Christ is also described in terms of scent, although with a more virtuous aspect. The Digby Mary Magdalene, preserved in one unique manuscript at Oxford's Bodleian Library, charts her journey from sinner to saint. Different scents in the play represent morality and immorality. The Virgin Mary is associated with the fragrances used in church such as frankincense and myrrh as well as medicinal perfumes including cinnabar, whereas Mary Magdalene is compared to a variety of smells that reflected her role as both saint and sinner: frankincense, gillyflowers, clary sage and musk.

Outdoor performances of religious dramas or miracle plays portraying stories from the Bible or scenes from the life of Christ were acted out by the various guilds of towns and cities. Because they traded in pleasant smells, the perfumers' guild might put on the story of Adam and Eve or perhaps the Annunciation. The tanners' guild of York, on the other hand, performed the fall of Lucifer and harrowing hell scenes, in keeping with the unpleasant odour of their industry – and also probably because of their easy access to those smells as dramatic aids.

## Miscellaneous Recipes
### A Perfume for Clothing

> Dissolve yellow sandalwood in rosewater and add one ounce of camphor. Use the mixture to perfume clothes, coats, and quilts.
> Abulcasis, *Al Tasreef Liman 'Ajaz 'Aan Al-Taleef* (The Clearance of Medical Science For Those Who Can Not Compile It), (*c.* AD 1000)

### Ghaliya

> Crush and sift one ounce of musk. Make sure to crush the musk gently so as not to be burnt. It is preferable if the musk is only sifted. Heat half an ounce of good quality ambergris. Leave it

on gentle heat. As it starts melting add a few drops of ben oil. Drain the mixture and add to the musk in a kettle. Make sure the ambergris is not very hot as it may ruin the musk. Crush the mixture and peel it with a gold plate do not use a copper or metal place so as not to ruin the mixture store the mixture in a gold or glass container.

Abulcasis, Al Tasreef

Note: The Islamic perfume Ghaliya was a mixture of musk, ambergris and ben oil. The prophet was said to have worn it on his beard. Abulcasis mentions a number of recipes for it, two of which are strictly for the caliphs and the elite. This is one of them.

## Perfumed Jewellery

Crush some saffron and some Arabic gum. Soak the Arabic gum in rosewater to soften and then mix a quarter of the Arabic gum with three quarters of saffron. Use the mixture to paint whatever jewels you want.

Abulcasis, Al Tasreef

## Syrup of Dried Roses

Take a *ratl* of dried roses, and cover with three *ratls* of boiling water, for a night, and leave it until they fall apart in the water. Press it and clarify it, take the clear part and add it to two *ratls* of white sugar, and cook all this until it is in the form of a syrup. Drink an *ûqiya* and a half of this with three of water. Its benefits: it binds the constitution, and benefits at the start of dropsy, fortifies the other internal organs, and provokes the appetite, God willing.

Anonymous, Andalusian cookbook (c. 1200s)

Note: The measures given are unclear. While they are common weights of Islamic origin for both dry and wet commodities in the medieval world, their weight varies over the period as well as from place to place.

## Scented Hair Powder

But when she combs her hair let her have this powder. Take some dried roses clove, nutmeg, watercress and galangal. Let all of these powdered be mixed with rose water. With this water let her sprinkle her hair and comb it with a comb dipped in the same water so that her hair will smell better. And let her make furrows in her hair and sprinkle on the above-mentioned powder and it will smell marvellously'.

Anonymous, *Trotula* (*c.* 1100s)

## Another Hair Powder

Also noblewomen should wear musk in their hair' or clove' or both but take care that it is not seen by anyone. Also the veil with which the head is tied should be put on with cloves and musk, nutmeg or other sweet smelling substances

*Trotula*

## Soap-like Mixture for Hand Washing

Together grind barley flour and bean flour thirty pennyweights of each; myrtle leaves, rose flower leaves, oregano, sweet marjoram, nabk, ten pennyweights each: sandalwood and costus five pennyweights of each and clove and musk and cardamom two pennyweights each. Knead the mixture with watermelon juice; make tablets and dry in the shade. Then crush the mixture add camphor and leave it to mature or you may incense it with aloeswood.

Abulcasis, *Al Tasreef*

# 5

# THE RENAISSANCE
## The Scented Stage, Printed Books and Pouncet Boxes

Dry roses put to the nose to smell do comfort the brayne [brain]
and the herte [heart] and quickeneth the spyryte [spirit].

*Banckes Herbal* (1525)

## Introduction

The cities of Florence and Venice saw the birth of the
Renaissance, a period of great cultural change in Europe during
the fifteenth centuries that, among many other things, fuelled
an enthusiasm for perfumes and encouraged their increasing use
across western Europe. During this time the city of Venice in
particular continued to thrive, as it had done towards the end
of the medieval period, as the most important centre for the
manufacture and trade in luxury goods, which of course included
scent.

At the beginning of the sixteenth century, perfume was more
likely to come in the form of a paste, a tablet or maybe a dry
powder rather than a liquid. However, as the century went
on liquid scent became much more the norm. In fact, even
at the beginning of the sixteenth century, although expensive
perfumes remained the prerogative of the social elite, flower

waters for everyday use were ubiquitous among the middle classes.

During the Renaissance, both men and women continued to wear scent and the elite set fashion trends. Perfume, with its erotic qualities, was also very much the stock in trade of the glamorous courtesans who charged men high prices for their services. These women were not without the means to purchase expensive scents themselves, but just like their counterparts in the classical world they would have expected to receive perfume in gifts from their clients.

The Renaissance was an era of strong odours. The *muschieri* or perfume makers of Venice were master craftsmen, selling scents based on musk, ambergris and cinnamon among other sought-after pungent ingredients. To match the high quality of Venetian fragrance, the glass factories of the city situated on Murano, a small group of interconnected islands in the Venetian lagoon, produced lavish coloured glass vessels. Now it was not only the exclusive contents that were coveted but the bottles themselves, which were prized for their artistry and their visible expression of wealth and status which carried throughout the courts of Europe. Even the ornate boxes used to store these decorative perfume bottles sometimes had moulded decoration known as *pasta di muschio*, basically a lead-based paint that was itself scented with musk.

As the sixteenth century progressed, other towns and cities became centres of perfume production in their own right. Chief among these new hubs of manufacture were the towns of Montpelier and Grasse in the south of France. Both grew an extensive range of flowers and fruits for the perfume market including oranges, jasmine and roses. In Grasse in particular, perfume manufacture developed alongside the glove making trade. Tanning had always been a smelly industry as urine was used to soften the leather during the process of making goods such as fans, shoes, gloves, bodices and belts. The leather industry therefore established a strong business connection with perfume makers as sweet fragrances were applied in order to counteract any lingering odours. The trendsetting ladies of the Italian Renaissance, and in particular Catherine de Medici (1519–1589), a member of the powerful Medici family of Florence and later Queen of France, set a fashion for wearing scented gloves. As a consequence, these quickly became the must-have fashion item among the upper crust.

Developments in transportation, chemistry and printing were key to the growth of perfume making at this time. Those who travelled far and wide discovered new sweet-smelling plants, learned from other cultures and facilitated the establishment of new trade routes. The expeditions of the Portuguese explorers Vasco da Gama (1469–1524) and Ferdinand Magellan (1480-1521) and the Italian Christopher Columbus (1451-1506) encouraged trade in vanilla, pepper, balsam, cardamom, sandalwood and cloves among other things. Columbus first encountered tobacco on his travels in the Americas, where he observed the indigenous people smoking and inhaling it in powder form. He made sure to bring back specimens of the plant, which would become a rather surprising perfume ingredient.

Creating a scent was not only a profession but a hobby for some, much as it was both a science and an art. Chemistry was now emerging from the more mystical discipline of alchemy as scientific experiment gained acceptance as a worthwhile profession for men and a legitimate hobby for wealthy ladies who had the time, means and opportunity to indulge in it. Not only were there new raw materials to experiment with, but there were developments in basic equipment as well. Instead of the copper of earlier times, stills used in this period were made of glass, which did not taint the scent. With the advent of the first printed books and a higher level of literacy, especially among women, expert knowledge and historic recipes began to circulate much more widely.

## Perfume: Morality and Immorality

> Moone and stares do obscure and darken the beames of the Sunne.
> So these (in as maner) palpable odours, fumes, vapours and smelles
> of Musks, Civets, Pomanders, Perfumes, Balmes and such like
> ascending to the briane doe rather darken and obscure the spirites
> and senses than either lighten them or comfort them in any way.
>
> Philip Stubbes, *The Anatomie of Abuses* (1583)

Perfume continued to serve functions both sacred and secular throughout the Renaissance. However, despite its increasing popularity, the ethics of its use, particularly in a religious context, remained a subject of hot debate. As if to illustrate the point, at her death in 1582, the body of the Spanish noblewoman Theresa of Avila was said to have exuded a strong smell of roses. This was viewed as proof of her sanctity in an echo of stories that had circulated in the medieval period. Ironically, given that this future saint was an ascetic who had abstained from all forms of indulgence – doubtless including perfume – she was unlikely to have smelled very pleasant in life.

Others, too, found it difficult to reconcile luxurious perfume with the exigencies of their faith. Indeed there was a resurgence of the idea that fragrance was an extravagance that encouraged depravity. Perfumes were among the items considered immoral and therefore burned by the Dominican friar, moralist and fanatic Savonarola (1452–1498), de facto ruler of Florence between 1494 and 1498, in what became known as the Bonfires of the Vanities. In his contemporary account of these bonfires the Italian historian Jacopo Nardi (1476–1563) recalled the destruction of 'an amazing multitude of such disgraceful statues and paintings, and also wigs and women's hair ornaments, bits of silk, cosmetics, orangeflower water, musk, perfumes of many sorts, and similar vanities...' The list goes on and on. As a result of such attitudes in the church, while the secular use of scent continued unabated, by the end of sixteenth century the use of incense had been confined to Catholic worship and was shunned by Protestants.

## Perfume: Ready-made and Homemade

While people could still buy the ingredients to make their own scent at home, the finished article was also on sale during the Renaissance. Apothecaries, the precursors of the modern chemist, sold ready-made perfumes as well as the ingredients to make them at home. Bucklersbury in London was famous for its apothecary shops selling exotic scented goods. The fact these apothecaries stocked scent was nothing out of the ordinary as the link between medicine and perfume remained close: the goods they were selling might have a dual purpose. In addition to such shops, itinerant pedlars and hawkers in the street also sold perfume alongside medicines, elixirs and other basic household items such as furniture wax. The city of Venice, as ever, appeared to be ahead of the game, with the *muschieri* establishing exclusive perfume boutiques.

Scent was much in demand and offered lucrative business opportunities, though competition was fierce. By the middle of the sixteenth century, according to the Italian playwright and satirist Pietro Aretino (1492–1556), in an attempt to control the trade in Venice it was stipulated that any street sellers must possess a valid licence to sell 'oils, unguents salves ... perfumed balls, musk, waters [and] civet'. Such restrictions existed in Florence too, with the guild of doctors and spice dealers controlling rights to sell soap and perfumes in the street.

Royalty in particular spent a fortune on scent. According to the household accounts of France's ruler Henri IV (1553–1610), in 1578 the king spent £96 just on violet powder to sprinkle on his clothes when they were stored in chests out of season.

In contrast, the raw ingredients to make perfume at home were not only on sale but might even be picked at little or no cost from one's own garden or the nearby hedgerows. Lavender was widely grown in sixteenth-century gardens and lavender water was a particularly popular homemade fragrance and remedy. Highly valued as a perfume for personal use too, lavender was applied to linen and sometimes used to scent soap. It could be mixed with other scents such as jasmine and with oils such as styrax, the latter to better fix and preserve the mixture and its scent. By the mid-sixteenth century lavender water was being distilled on country estates across England, and by 1568 the plant was being grown on a commercial scale in Hertfordshire and Surrey.

## Santa Maria Novella

Tucked away in a relatively quiet street in Florence, Santa Maria Novella may be the world's oldest surviving pharmacy. Founded as a monastery by Dominican friars back in the thirteenth century, it first came to the aid of the city during the outbreak of plague in the fourteenth century. The Dominicans were an order dedicated to poverty and charity, which goes to reinforce the idea that the perfumed waters they made and offered for sale were intended primarily as cures for illness and not luxurious items for personal adornment. Being known as an outlet for medical cures based on scent meant that the monks, or at least their precious products, escaped a roasting in Savonarola's bonfires. Under the patronage of Catherine de' Medici, business flourished at Santa Maria Novella. Indeed, the monks created a perfume especially for her majesty on her marriage to the King of France, naming it Acqua Della Regina (Water of the Queen). The scent was a mixture of bergamot, lemon, lavender and rosemary.

Remarkably, apart from a brief period at the very beginning of the seventeenth century, the manufacture and sale of fragrances at Santa Maria Novella has continued uninterrupted to the present day. Among other scented goods one can still purchase their rosewater, which is now recognised as a toner and a perfume in its own right but was originally used as a disinfectant to counteract the fourteenth-century outbreak of the plague.

## Perfume in Print

As mentioned above, the advent of the printing press saw recipes for perfumes become much more widely accessible – for those who could read or knew somebody who could, at least. More specifically, a particular genre of book, later referred to as Books of Secrets, fuelled and preserved interest in a number of topics including fragrances. Initially these books were printed in Italian, then French and Spanish, and later in English. They were basically self-help manuals, often containing instructions for everything from how to cook a chicken to making a scented powder to sprinkle on one's clothing. The word 'secret' was intended to give the idea that these texts divulged some sort of ancient wisdom, and in a sense they did. The recipes were in fact based on a combination of traditional knowledge, folklore and the contents of personal family housekeeping records, and were sometimes cleverly attributed to well-known aristocratic ladies in a historic equivalent of today's celebrity endorsement.

Predictably it was Venice that witnessed the printing of the first of these Books of Secrets on the art of perfume making, namely *Venusta*, penned by the writer and artist Eustachio Celebrino (1490–1535) and printed in La Serenissima in 1526. Around this time, in 1544, the physician and naturalist Pietro Andrea Mattioli (1501–1577) translated Dioscurides' seminal treatise on pharmacology from the Greek into Italian and proliferated knowledge of subjects associated with scent. One of the most well-known works on perfume from this period is *Notandissimi Secreti de L'Arte Profumatoria* (The Very Noble Secrets of Perfumery Art) by Giovanni Rosetti, first printed in Venice in 1555. The text gives detailed recipes and formulas for making perfumes, perfumed waters, scented lotions, fragrant cosmetics and soaps. There are recipes for air fresheners or room scents in the book too. The book also specifies that some scents were for use not only at different times of year (understandable given limited availability) but even at different times of the day. Rosetti's book alone contains more than three hundred perfume recipes, among them a recipe for soap in which rosewater, powdered cherry kernels, storax, musk and spike oil were added to a pound of white soap, the older the better. Once the ingredients are mixed, Rosetti instructs the reader to 'make into little soaps using moulds or from them into little balls. Dry them in the shade. Wrap in cotton and put in a box.'

*I secreti della Signora Isabella Cortese* (The secrets of Signora Isabella Cortese), published in 1561, is another example of this genre and is supposedly the work of an Italian noblewoman. She directs her advice for fine musk oil at 'every great lady'. However, not all the perfume recipes that circulated at this time were intended for female use. There were scented products aimed exclusively at male personal care too; in the secrets of Alessio Piedmontese – thought to be a pseudonym of the Venetian polymath Girolamo Ruscelli (1550-1566) – we find the following recipe for beard oil:

> To make oile Imperial, to perfume the haire or beard of a man, to rub his handes or gloves with, and to put also into the lye or water, wherein princes or great mens clothes be washed: and this oyle may a man make with cost enough, and also with little charge and expense.

The ingredients for the above scent included rosewater, Damask rose oil, cloves, cinnamon, gum Arabic, musk and civet.

Books of Secrets not only spread the knowledge of how to make a perfume but sometimes included recipes for less expensive scents that might be useful on a daily basis. Although the best perfumes remained the prerogative of the rich, these printed books allowed the less well-off the opportunity to emulate their wealthy counterparts by making their own cheaper versions of exclusive scents. Sir Hugh Platt (1552–1608), in his work *Delights for Ladies*, acknowledged the demand for reasonably priced products, describing a water for washing one's hands as 'very cheap ... it is composed of water, lavender, cloves, iris powder and benjamin'.

## *Herbs, Hygiene and Handwashing*

> I met with wagones, Cartes, & Horses full loden with yong barnes,
> for fear of the blacke Pestilence, with their boxes of Medicens and
> sweete perfume. O God, how fast did they run by hundreds, and
> were afraid of eche other for feare of smityng.
>
> William Bullein, *Bulleins Bulwarke* (1562)

Throughout the Renaissance, there prevailed a belief that scent was effective against the spread of disease. Outbreaks of plague continued to sweep Europe and sweet-smelling flowers, aromatic herbs and pungent animal excretions were deemed important in the containment of these pandemics as well as the prevention and treatment of diseases in general. The term 'essential oil' was used for the first time in the sixteenth century by physician and alchemist Paracelsus (1493–1541) to describe the effective component of a drug. In 1562, physician and cleric William Bullein (c. 1515–1576), quoted above, published *Bulleins Bulwarke (regarding defence against sickness)*. He believed in the therapeutic power of plants and recorded various methods of perfuming linen, clothes and other personal belongings in an effort to promote cleanliness and good health.

While stronger substances like arsenic, ammonia and quicklime were used as disinfectants, gentler scents might be applied to items that were touched, such as furniture. Cinnamon, rose, civet, orange blossom and musk were taken internally or applied to the surface of the body as remedies or cures. Naturalist William Turner (1508–1568) in his *Newe Herbal*, published in 1551 and thus the first printed herbal in the English language, stated, 'I judge that the flowers of lavender quilted in a cap and dayly worne are good for all diseases of the head that come of a cold cause and that they comfort the braine very well.' The French astrologer and physician Nostradamus (1503–1566), known more for his apparent ability to predict the future than for his interest in scent, favoured labdanum not only for its lovely perfume but because he believed that there was 'nothing better for protecting one against infection in times of pestilence'. He added that 'it cheers up humans and strengthens the heart and the brain'. The *Grete Herbal*, published in 1529, noted that rosemary is 'a comfort in its smell'. Fragrances, then, were still very much a multipurpose remedy for a wide variety of complaints.

Bathing as a matter of routine was not popular. The experience of the plague had made people very afraid of water; they saw it as a carrier of disease, and feared that a bath could easily result in a chill and subsequently a deadly fever. In fact, women and men bathed probably less in this period than they had done in medieval times. Instead of bathing, both sexes washed parts of their body (particularly the extremities) to prevent the smell of sweat, often using rosewater mixed with white lead, salt, coriander and sedge. Keeping one's linen underclothes clean with soap remained vital in the fight against disease, but this product was still extremely caustic and malodorous so had little contact with the body. However, soap for personal hygiene did become more popular around the middle of the sixteenth century. In one anonymous Venetian recipe book dating from 1555, the writer suggests adding 'benzoin, storax or frankincense or indeed any other scent that you favour' to basic hard soap made from soda ash. This would certainly have produced a nicer smell than basic soap made of sheep fat and pot ash. Adding your own fragrance to soap at home was also much less expensive than buying high-end Castile soap, which by now was available to those in Britain who could afford it.

The one exception to public antipathy towards bathing was the steam bath, also known as a vaporary or a moist stove. Taking this sort of bath was believed to be beneficial for both sexes as a medical treatment. The purpose of the steam bath was to sweat out a disease with healing aromatics. Women's steam baths were scented with herbs such as jasmine, lavender, hyssop, bay leaves, comfrey and rosemary, and Sir Hugh Platt advised that 'such proportion of sweet hearbes and of such a kind as shall be most appropriate for your infirmitie ... will breathe so sweet and warme a vapour upon your body as that you shall sweat temperately'.

Perfumes were also used to manage birthing pains. One Florentine manuscript advises, 'Take one quattrino of crushed weeds and one quattrino of crushed incense and heat over an open fire with a lid. When the lid is taken off the smoke given off helps pain.' Scent was also used when trying to conceive by perfuming the woman's genitals with aloeswood. According to the sixteenth-century physician Giovanni Marinello in his 1562 work *Gli ornamenti delle donne* (Cosmetics for Ladies), a room scented with perfume would encourage the conception of a male child, that all-important son and heir.

Many claims were made for scent on the more superficial level of preserving youth and beauty. According to *Banckes Herbal* (1525), one should 'make thee a box of the wood of rosemary and smell to it and it shall preserver thy youth'. An impossible claim no doubt, but scented cosmetic products like mouthwashes made from herbs such as peppermint, thyme and vinegar could certainly conceal bad breath and the smell of decaying teeth, which often worsened as a person aged. Other fragranced products such as scented hair powders were as likely to attract vermin as they were to make one appear more attractive.

## Perfuming the Home

> Of Rosemary take the flowers and put them in thy chest among the clothes or thy books and mothes shall not destroy them.
> Thomas Dawson, *The Good Housewife's Jewell* (1585)

Managing unwanted pests using aromatic herbs as cookery writer Thomas Dawson (1585–1620) recommends above was but one of the many domestic applications for scent at the time. In his *Treasurie of Commodius Receipts* (1578) author John Partridge includes recipes to perfume gloves, chests and cupboards, scent for the fire to perfume and fumigate the house as well as a violet powder specifically for woollen clothes and furs. He claims southernwood (in French the word for southernwood is *garderobe*, meaning 'clothes protector') deters moths and was laid among stored items of clothing. To ensure a good night's sleep, pillows were stuffed with lavender and a mixture of peppermint, cloves and rose petals.

Rooms were sprinkled with scent using silver containers that resembled small watering cans with holes for spraying the scent. Sometimes they were crafted in other shapes, with surviving examples including a lemon-shaped version. Perforated perfume burners were also commonly found in bedrooms. Also known as charcoal burners, fuming pots or stink pots, they worked by heating scented pastilles to give off a pleasant odour. There was scented soap in bedchambers as well as perfumed lamps. *Oiselets de Chypre* (Cyprus fledglings) were similar to pomanders but in the shape of small birds, made of cloth decorated with real feathers and stuffed with aromatics such as oak moss, cypress, iris root, labdanum, storax and almond. They were hung from walls and ceilings. Their popularity began to grow in the 1520s, and they are depicted in works of art and recorded in the account books of the wealthy from this period.

If harsher measures were required, for instance in the wake of a serious outbreak of illness, a professional fumigator might be hired who would seal the windows and doors while he walked from room to room with a steaming pan of aromatics, wafting smoke in all directions.

## Herb Strewing

> Where's the cook? Is supper ready, the house trimmed, rushes strewed, cobwebs swept?
> William Shakespeare, *The Taming of the Shrew* (1590–94)

In the above quotation, and indeed elsewhere in his plays, William Shakespeare (1564–1616) alludes to the practice of strewing floors. Helpfully, the poet and farmer Thomas Tusser (1524–1580) in *Five Hundred Points of Good Husbandrie*, his gardening book from 1557, goes into more detail, giving us a list of herbs used for this purpose. They include basil, camomile, costmary, cowslips, daisies, fennel, germander, hyssop, lavender, lemon balm, marjoram, maudeline, mints, pennyroyal, roses, sage, savory, tansy and violet. Clearly there was plenty of choice.

In *Gerard's Herbal*, author John Gerard (1545–1612), a botanist and owner of a large herb garden in London, noted that Elizabeth I particularly appreciated meadowsweet strewn on the floors of her chambers. Herbalist and botanist John Parkinson (1567–1650) in his 1640 work *The Theatre of Plants*, remarks that 'Queen Elizabeth of famous memory did more desire it [meadowsweet] than any other sweet herbe to strew her chambers with'. The Dutch traveller Levimus Lemnius (1505-1568) records in his diary that when he visited England in 1560 'chambers and parlours strawed all over with fresh herbs refreshed me: their nosegays finally intermingled with sundry sorts of fragrant floures in their bedchambers and privy rooms with comfortable smell cheered me up and entirely delighted all my senses'. No doubt encountering bad smells was one of the perils of travelling, and we can be sure that not all travellers' lodgings were quite so fragrant.

## At the Table: Dining Etiquette, Scented Food and Drink

Clean the flower and, when washed, crush it and squeeze it well with your hands; and then wash it in clean water, moving the water until the orange blossom has become sweet. And when it is sweet, take two parts of the flower and one of clarified sugar high temperature, and another of clarified honey. And once it is cold, add the orange blossom that has been very well-squeezed with your hands, and mix it well, and put in a little musk dissolved in scented water.

Orange blossom conserve recipe,
*Manual de Mugeres* (1500s)

By the mid-sixteenth century it was the practice in well-off households for table linen to be scented. In his *Dialogues*, Petro Aretino (1492–1596) mentions 'perfuming a cloth with lavender more pungent than the muskrat makes'. The tables in the houses of the elite were also loaded with scented food and perfumed drinks. The poor might even be 'privileged' to watch the elite eating and so get sight, and of course smell, of their voluptuous food. Wines and teas were scented with lavender or marigold and there were syrups, honeys, vinegars, oils, and conserves scented and flavoured with roses or perhaps sweet violets. Thomas Lupton in his *A Thousand Notable Things of Sundry Sortes*, published in 1579, advises, 'Wine will be pleasant in taste and in savour and in colour it will much please thee if an orange or a lemon stickt around with cloaves be hanged within the vessel that it touch not the wyne and so the wyne will be preserved from foystimnes: so preservative.'

Desserts like sorbet were sprinkled with musk and amber. Even the preparation of grilled meat might require scented ingredients. Bartolomeo Platina (1421–1481), author of *De Honesta Voluptate et Valetudine* (1474), the first printed cookbook, includes the following instructions in his recipe for roast chicken: 'You will roast a chicken after it has been well plucked, cleaned and washed; and after roasting it, put it into a dish before it cools off and pour over it either orange juice or verjuice with rosewater, sugar and well-ground cinnamon, and serve it to your guests.'

Bowls of rosewater still took pride of place on the tables of the aristocracy as most people continued to eat with their hands. In order to provide a pleasant backdrop to one's meal, at court and in the best houses, fountains spouted scented water. Again, according to Platina, in the winter months when fresh flowers were not so readily available the host must ensure that in their dining room 'the air should be redolent of perfumes'. For the upper classes, at least, the whole act of dining must have been quite a stimulating olfactory experience.

## Scented Clothing and Sweet Bags

Take of Ireos. ii. ounces, of Calamus aromaticus. iii. quarters of an
ounce, of Cipres, or gallingal, of Spiknale, of Rose leues dried, of
ech a quarter of an ounce, of cloues of Spyke: or Lauender flowres,
of each halfe an ounce: of Nigella romana, a quarter of an ounce:
of Beniamin, or Storax calimit: of each halfe an ounce. Let them
be all finely beaten, and serced, then take two or three graynes of
Musk disloue it in rose water, and sprinckell the water vpon the
powder, and turne it vp and downe in the sprincklyng, tyl it haue
drunke vp the water, when it is dry, kepe it in bagges of sylke.

John Partridge, *The Treasurie of*
*Commodious Conceits* (1573)

It was an onerous task to keep heavy dresses and layers of
underclothes clean and smelling fresh, but it wasn't only women
who had to consider such things; men for their part wore scented
waistcoats, doublets, belts and shoes. Therefore, extensive use was
made of perfumed sachets known as sweet bags which were sewn
into clothes to help camouflage unpleasant odours. The contents
of these small bags included rose powder, civet and ambergris
mixed with orris root; the latter was added to prolong the smell.
These sweet bags were a welcome upgrade from the practice of
merely sprinkling powder directly onto clothes in storage.

While John Partridge recommends violet powder for women's
clothes and furs, he suggests a sweet powder comprised of red roses,
marjoram and musk for linens. Partridge stresses the importance
of collecting the ingredients when fresh and, with special reference
to the roses, in clement weather: 'In the soomer time father red
roses in fair wether so sonne as they be blowne and opened.' Sweet
bags were also deemed a suitable gift even for a queen. As a New
Year present in the year 1561–2, one Mr William Huggyns gave
Elizabeth I 'a great swete bag of tapphata … embroidered with
Venice gold and pearles'. Given the quality of the bag itself, we can
only imagine the expensive scents it might have held.

## Accessories; Gloves, Handkerchiefs and Fans

> The gloves must be delicate
> And very little worn
> Indeed oiled thoroughly
> And lastingly perfumed
> With exciting odours
> You know of balsamic resin
> With fragrant oil of balm.
>
> Castilian poem (1511)

William Bullein in his *Bullwarke* advocated perfuming not only clothes and linen but also one's personal belongings in general. Certainly the smell of leather was too much for some, and to counteract the lingering bad odour from the manufacturing and treatment processes fans made of leather were scented with delicate toilette waters such as orange water. As a result, fluttering a fan was also a very acceptable way of freshening the surrounding air.

Scented gloves in particular became not only fashionable but an expensive commodity, a visible (and sensory) sign of the owner's wealth. The importance of the hand in common gesture – and, more specifically, at the first meeting of a betrothed couple – meant the glove as well as the hand inside it was vital to first impressions. Leather gloves were perfumed with a variety of scents including exotic jasmine. An Italian phrasebook dating from 1578 and compiled by one John Florio (1553–1625), who was among other things a translator, poet, and royal language tutor at the court of James I, contains numerous phrases regarding gloves including how to ask whether they were well perfumed: 'These Gloves, are they well perfumed? ... Who hath perfumed them? ... I will haue them perfumed.'

Scented gloves were considered appropriate diplomatic gifts. The Duke of Tuscany and his duchess received a number of pairs of gloves from the Spanish ambassador to the Medici court. Isabella D'este (1474–1539), Marchioness of Mantua and a leading figure both culturally and politically, gave gifts of perfume, scented gloves and other objects to friends and those she favoured. Isabella also tried to ban prostitutes from wearing perfumed gloves as she considered that it was not in keeping with their status.

Ornate scented handkerchiefs also became very popular under Catherine de' Medici in France and Elizabeth I in England as both ladies appreciated them and therefore set a trend. The handkerchief when dipped in perfume had the advantage of retaining its scent well and was useful for holding over the nose when one encountered bad or even potentially dangerous smells. Handkerchiefs were also given as presents and could be of sufficient value to be listed in wills and inventories of a person's possessions. The handkerchief could be carried in a sweet bag when not in use, though it was perfectly acceptable to have the item on show and close to hand.

## Portable Perfume: Pomanders, Casting Bottles and Pouncet Boxes

> To make a pomander; 2 ounces of labdanum; of Benjamin and storax one ounce; musk six graines; ambergrease six graines; of calamus aromaticus and lignum aloes of each the weight of a groat; beat all these together in a hot mortar and with a hot pestle until they come to a paste; then wet your hands with rosewater and rowle up the paste suddenly.
>
> Hugh Platt, *Delights for Ladies* (1594)

The beginning of the sixteenth century was the heyday of the pomander, which had grown more sophisticated since the medieval era. In the first place, other scents had been added to the common mixtures, including camphor, sandalwood and myrrh combined with rosewater. Scents like these are known to have some antiseptic properties, so their addition may have improved the pomander's effectiveness as preventative medicine. Combating illness was, of course, the primary purpose of the pomander, though it was also considered an effective defence against magic. While the practice of carrying the pomander on a chain that hung from a belt or necklace continued, the design as well as the scent became more intricate. There were pomanders that divided into segments just like an orange, with each segment containing a different perfume. Although the traditional shape was a round ball, pomanders also began to come in many different designs in this period including quite outlandish examples such as skulls and ships.

The end of the sixteenth century saw the decline of the pomander as liquid perfume became more common. Pomanders were replaced with bottles designed not only to contain scent but also to be worn and displayed, again as a symbol of wealth and status. Made of gold or silver and studded with jewels, these objects could make quite an impression. A particular type of bottle known as a casting bottle had perforated holes to allow scent to be easily and discreetly sprinkled onto one's clothes even when out and about.

Another container that became fashionable at this time was the pouncet box. This was made of silver or gold and had a perforated lid (the word pouncet means pierced). Inside there would be a small sponge soaked in weak vinegar. The holes in the lid allowed the scent to escape into the air. These boxes originated in Britain and were considered a luxury item, favoured by both men and women in the sixteenth century and into the middle of the seventeenth. It was part of court etiquette to hold one's pouncet box to one's nose, but men could be ridiculed for this; in Shakespeare's *Henry IV Part 1*, Henry 'Hotspur' Percy gives this description of a captive lord: 'He was perfumed like a milliner, And twixt his finger and his thumb he held a pouncet box, which, ever and anon, he gave his nose and took't away again.'

## Perfumed Jewellery

We know that rosaries were originally made from dried rosebuds or beads made from resin, hence the name. In the sixteenth century these were turned into necklaces, pendants and bracelets. The widow of Cesare Borgia, Charlotte of Albret (1480–1514), had rosaries made in the form of enamelled, pierced gold beads for holding and emitting scent. Some women wore a larger pomander bead in the centre of a necklace with smaller beads filled with spices to ward off illness or conceal body odour. Mary, Queen of Scots wore scented jewellery and is said to have favoured a particular string of scented beads. There also exist lockets housing small pieces of perfume-soaked cloth dating from the sixteenth century.

Rings with a thicker hoop and with a valve at the back were another form of scented jewellery. The ring would first be doused in perfume with the valve pressed flat. When the valve was released the scent would be drawn up into the ring ready to be released with the minimum of pressure in a spray as required. Sometimes these rings were rumoured to hold poison disguised as scent. According to tradition, the plotters who attempted to poison William the Silent (1533–1584), Prince of Orange, in 1582 used a ring. Poison-laden scent was not a new method of murder, of course, having featured in connection with other fashion items. In Christopher Marlowe's drama *The Massacre at Paris*, first performed in 1593, a pair of scented gloves are identified as a murder weapon.

## Scent in the Theatre

Not only could scent be central to plot as in Marlowe's play, but in popular sixteenth-century drama it was very much part of the production. Actual scent was used as a prop or element of stagecraft in the theatre at this time. According to daily accounts of the court for 1 January 1573, in producing a play performed by the children of Windsor Chapel, apothecary Robert Moorer 'provided sugar, musk comfits, corianders, clove comfits, cinnamon comfits, rose water, spice water, ginger comfits … all which served for flakes of ice and hail-stones in the masque of Janus, the rose water sweetened the balls made for snowballs'.

According to *Hall's Chronicle*, in November 1527 Henry VIII made use of a perfumed fountain during the interlude in a drama performed in honour of the French ambassador. The latter was surely impressed by the 'fayre lady out of whose breasts ran abundantly water of miraculous delicious savour'.

Scent also served to camouflage the stench emanating from the audience. The common folk watching the action occupied the standing room directly in front of the stage and were generally crowded together. They were known as groundlings but also, reflecting their odour in the summer months, as stinkards. The contemporary playwright John Marston (1576–1634) described the poor as 'choked with the stench of garlic' in reference to their daily diet.

## Shakespeare and the Meaning of Fragrance

> There' s rosemary, that's for remembrance.
> Pray you, love, remember.
> And there is pansies, that's for thoughts ...
> There's fennel for you, and columbines.
> There's rue for you, and here's some for me.
> ...I would give you some violets,
> But they withered all when my father died.
>
> William Shakespeare, *Hamlet*

Long before the Victorians made the language of flowers popular, in the composition of Ophelia's bouquet above, in the mischief that ensues in the *Midsummer Night's Dream* and in the horror and tragedy of *Hamlet* and *Macbeth*, flowers and their scents were imbued with meaning. The Bard used perfume to help explain the action on stage and tell the story. He favoured realism and accuracy too where plants were concerned, with fragrances appropriate to the seasons in which the play was set; for example, in *The Winter's Tale* the rogue and jack-of-all-trades Autolycus mentions daffodils as he sings about the coming of spring.

Many of the characters in Shakespeare's plays have some connection with scent: the tragic Ophelia, the beautiful Titania and the distressed Lady Macbeth are but three of a multitude of possible examples. Indeed, perfume by its omnipresence almost seems to be a character in its own right in Shakespearean drama. Cleopatra's perfume in *Antony and Cleopatra* bewitches Antony in the tradition of the original story, and represents power and desire. There is much floral symbolism in *A Midsummer Night's Dream*, too, where Titania's bed is made of perfumed herbs and flowers. *The Winter's Tale* and *The Merry Wives of Windsor* both make mention of perfumed gloves; in the former those gloves are pronounced 'as sweet as damask roses'.

In the so-called 'Scottish Play', Lady Macbeth finds the stench of blood and death on her hands so strong that even using perfumes from Arabia, long considered the best and the most expensive, cannot remove it. Benedick, a lovesick gentleman in *Much Ado about Nothing*, rubs himself with civet; his perfume is a clue to his state of mind.

## The Rich and Famous: Catherine, Isabella, Henry and Elizabeth

In 1547, on the occasion of her marriage to the fourteen-year-old Henri II, Catherine de' Medici became Queen of France. The new queen brought to her new home the knowledge of perfumes that she had acquired in her native Italy. In the south of France flower production grew, fuelled by competition to meet the demand for fragrances. Catherine's personal perfumer, Rene de Florentin, accompanied her from Florence and served her well in her new home. Born Renato Bianco at the turn of the century, he had been abandoned at birth and as a consequence brought up by the apothecary monks at Santa Maria Novella, where he absorbed their vast knowledge of fragrances. Catherine was of course involved in the production of her favourite scents and was famously rumoured to have used poison, and while there is no proof that she did so, the fact that Rene de Florentin sold poison alongside perfumes and cosmetics in his shop near Notre Dame Cathedral did nothing to quash these stories either.

Not so involved but nevertheless a devotee of fragrance, Henry VIII had his clothes scented with lavender and orange flower water. Later, his bedchamber would be heavily scented with rosewater as he lay on his deathbed; something had to be done to counteract the putrid smell coming from his leg sores. Elizabeth I wore perfumed clothes as she, like many others, did not take a bath very often; in fact she is thought to have restricted her bathing to twice a year. Perhaps this was in view of her own brush with serious illness, having been smitten with smallpox when young. However, allegedly the queen was very sensitive to smell. In 1573, Edward de Vere (1550–1604), 17th Earl of Oxford, brought her a gift of 'perfumed gloves, sweet bags and other pleasant things'. A pair of these scented gloves from Italy survives to this day in the Bodleian Library in Oxford. According to Bernardino de Mendoza (1540–1604), a Spanish writer and military man, a present of perfumed gloves could gain the queen's favour: 'I am told by a person in the Palace that, even in the matter of giving me audience readily, the Queen has been considerably influenced by the gloves and perfumes which I gave her when I arrived.'

The queen's wardrobe accounts detail expenditure on the perfuming of her clothing. We know that in 1579 eight dresses and four fans were fragranced with musk, civet and ambergris. Earlier in 1572 the instructions to her wardrobe master included the perfuming of two pairs of shoes. The queen had perfumes for all seasons but favoured toilet water scented with marjoram. Her chambers were scented with burning incense and her ladies carried pomanders with them. The wardrobe accounts suggest the purchase of staggering amounts of ingredients such as orris powder for use in her private rooms. Her leather laced bodices were also scented. The queen received many gifts of scent as part of New Year tradition, in 1561 receiving among other things 'a little round mounte of golde to conteyne a pomaunder in it', two sweet bags, a 'box of pyne comfetts musked' and 'a spice plate, with a cover'.

## Nostradamus

Though better remembered for his prophecies, Nostradamus (1503–1566) was a respected sixteenth-century doctor and healer. His book of elixirs was originally published in French in 1552 and contains a wide variety of recipes for aromatic pastes and oils, scents for rosary or paternoster beads, sweet waters and fragrant powders. He extols the virtues of roses 'to all aromatic mixtures are added roses which are the best things for imparting scent although they lose it on account of their subtle and delicate substance'. What he lacks in precise measurements Nostradamus makes up for in the details of preparation, referring to earthenware pots, the value of fat from a pig slaughtered just the day before, and the importance of using Florentine violets and the best, sweet-smelling apples.

## Recipes: A Selection
### Soap

> Take soap that has been in the sun and purged with a little oil of benzoin and mix you can use oil of storax or oldano (frankincense) or another kind of scent you like and mal yur balls or wash balls...
>
> Alexis of Piedmont, *Book of Secrets* (1555)

### Sweet Water for Linen

> Three pounds of Rose water, cloves, cinnamon, Sauders [sandalwood], 2 handful of the flowers of Lavender, lette it stand a moneth to still in the sonne, well closed in a glasse; Then destill it in Balneo Marial. It is marvellous pleasant in savour, a water of wondrous swetenes, for the bedde, whereby the whole place, shall have a most pleasaunt scent.
>
> William Bullein, *Bulleins Bulwarke* (1562)

## Musk Soap

Take stronge lye made of chalk, and six pounde of stone chalk: iiii, pounde of Deere Suet, and put them in the lye; in an earthen potte, and mingle it well, and kepe it the space of forty daies, and mingle and [styr? fyr?] it, iii, or, iiii times a daye, tyll it be consumed, and that, that remayneth, vii, or, viii, dayes after, then you muste put a quarter of an ounce of Muske, and when you have done so, you must [sty?re] it, and it wyll smell of Musk.

John Partridge, *The Treasurie of Commodious Conceits* (1573)

## A Perfume for Chestes and Cubbords: And also for Gloues.

Take Benjamin and Storax, of each one ounce, Labdanum, and Fusses, of each a quarter of an ounce, halfe a Dramme of Ciuet. If you burne it for Chestes, or Cubbordes, heate it in a hot Morter. If it be for Gloues, boyle it and put it to Rose water

John Partridge, *The Treasurie of Commodious Conceits* (1573)

## White Musk Soap

Take soap scraped or grated, as much as you need the which (when you have well steeped and tempered in rose water) leave it eight days in the sun: Then you shall add to it an ounce of the water or milk of Macaleb [Prumus maheleb], twelve grains of musk, and six grains of civet, and reduce all together into the form and manner of a hard paste, you shall make of this very excellent balls.

Girolamo Ruscelli, *The secretes of the reuerende Maister Alexis of Piemount* (1558)

## Perfumed Tablets

Two pounds of rose water and a pound of citrus blossom water a pound of benzoin and half of balsam an ounce of amber and half of musk a quarter of civet musk all together and ground put it with the water in a flask put the flask on the fire over some embers stir with a stick and cook until in reduced three parts from one and when it reduced remove the paste from that and make into tablets if you wish tablets and if not keep this as a paste.

Anonymous, Manual de Mugeres (1500s)

## Rose-scented Tablets

Take a pound of roses without the flower heads, and seven ounces of ground benzoin. Put the roses to soak in musk water for a night. Remove these roses afterwards and thoroughly squeeze out the water, and grind them with the benzoin. And when grinding, put with it a quarter of amber and another of civet [musk]. And after [they are] ground, make your tablets and put each one between two rose leaves, and dry them away from the sun.

Anonymous, Manual de Mugeres (1500s)

## Unction for Combing Hair

Two pounds of very fat and very well-blended bacon cut into small pieces. And put it in a stew-pot, put with it a fourth part of head lye and four maravedís of alhovas, and a fourth of linseed, and a fourth of barberry, and a (fourth) of calamus gum, and another (fourth) of bastard saffron (safflower), and another (fourth) of rough cumin. Put the stew-pot on the fire with all these things, and once the bacon comes apart, strain it with another large stew-pot and throw in three or four lizards. And put the lid on the stew-pot very well. Cook it in the oven and, when cooked, strain it and keep it in a bottle. And comb your hair with it.

Anonymous, Manual de Mugeres (1500s)

## Scented (and Medicated Soap)

To make well scented soap against scabies. Take strong lye, in which you will do a little bit of salt, and let it well dissolve together; then take a little rosewater, and the juice of lemons, and also much of the mentioned salted lye. Add into this white soap broken and cut up small, and a little clove powder; let this stand until it becomes like dough, which you stir with a stick in a deep dish, then put it in the sun until the mentioned soap becomes hard, so that you can lightly make balls, of the size you like. After you made them, let them dry, and use them every morning to wash the hands, and you will have no more worry of the scabies, because when you do this before, you won't bother it.

Anonymous, *T Bouck va Wondre* (1513)

## Sweet Water

To make a sweet water of the best kind: Ingredients a thousand damask roses lavender, mace, cloves and fresh water mixed and kneaded over four days.

Hugh Platt, *Delightes for Ladies* (1594)

## Soap to Keep Hands White and Soft

Take some yew root, scrape it without washing it and dry it in the shade. Next, pulverize it and take four ounces of it, one ounce of wheat flour, six dracms of ground pine-nut kernels, two ounces of almond kernels from which the oil has been well pressed, one ounce and a half of clean bitter-orange pips, two ounces each of oil of tartar and sweet almond oil and a half drachm of musk. Grind these up into the finest possible powder and for every ounce of this powder add half an ounce of Florentine violet roots. Next take a further half pound of yew root and let it soak overnight in good-quality rose-water or bitter-orange blossom-water. Squeeze the water and roots thoroughly and knead the exuded slime with the other ingredients. Add the musk and make the mixture into globes or round balls. Dry them and when you want to use them, take one in your hand, pour water over it and rub your hands with it and they will become white and tender and soft. Gaetan soap, however, is excluded, though others do use it, for although it whitens the hands, it also makes them rough and dry or chapped, because it is made from a strong, sharp lye, namely from the chalk of ordinary silica ashes, from which glass has been made, and the ashes of burnet tartar. Gaetan soap has, however, been made from chalk and burnt tartar for a very long while and, although that soap is prepared from this lye and from ordinary olive oil, it still makes the hands very rough. Our composition for soap, however, is very gentle and pleasant, for only mild substances are used in it and even if the hands are already hard, after using it two or three times they will become as gentle and soft as if they were the hands of a young girl of ten.

Nostradamus, *The Elixirs
of Nostradamus* (1552)

## Teeth Cleaner

Also take the timber thereof [rosemary] and burn it to coals and make powder thereof and put it into a linen cloth and rub they teeth therewith and if there be any worms therein it shall slay them and keep thy teeth from all evils.

*Banckes Herbal* (1525)

## Musk-scented Soap

Take a half ounce of calamita storax, and an ounce of benzoin, and a quarter ounce of liquid storax and a quarter ounce of sallow sandalwood. All this pulverized and well re-soaked in musk-scented water, mix together with a half pound of white soap and with one ounce of deer marrow. And cut everything up very well, sprinkling it with musk-scented water and you will cut it up until it has drunk one ounce of musk-scented water. And then you will bring together with this the weight of a dinero [a silver coin] of amber, and a grain of musk dissolved in a little of this water. And you will mix this very well in a stone mortar in the by whipping.

Anonymous, *Manual de Mugeres* (1500s)

## Deodorant

Take two pounds of rosewater an ounce of white lead four drams of slat one of azisi and two of coriander sedge and one of benzoin. Pound these things all together boiling a little then cool. Bathe whatever areas have the stench and you may then delight in the soft fragrance.

Giovanni Marinello, *Gli ornamenti delle Donne* (1562)

## 'A Fumigation for a Presse, and Clothes that no Moth shall Breed there in'

Take of the wood of Cipres, or of Ieniper, of Rasemary dried, of Storax Calamit, of Beniamin, of Cloues, a like waight beaten all in to pouder, then take of ye powder of Wormwood leaues dried: as muche as all ye others, mixe them well together, cast therof vpon a Chafyngdish of coles and set it in your pres and shut it close, & thus do ofttimes tyll you have well seasoned your Presse or Coffer.

John Partridge, *The Treasurie of Commodious Conceits* (1573)

## Of Rosemary

Take the Flowers, and put the in thy Chest, among thy clothes or among thy Bokes, and Mothes shall not destroy them.

John Partridge, *The Treasurie of Commodious Conceits* (1573)

## A Violet powder for Wullun Clothes and Furres

Take of Ireos. ii. ounces, of Calamus aromaticus. iii. Quarters of an ounce, of Cipres, or gallingal, of Spiknale, of Rose leues dried, ofech a quarter of an ounce, of cloues of Spyke: or Lauender Flowres, of each halfe an ounce: of Nigella ro|mana, a quarter of an ounce: of Beniamin, of Storax calimit: of each halfe an ounce. Let them be all finely beaten, and serced, then take two or three graynes of Musk disloue it in rose water, and sprinc|kell the water vpon the powder, and turne it vp and downe in the sprincklyng, tyl it haue drunke vp the water, when it is dry, kepe it in bagges of sylke.

John Partridge, *The Treasurie of Commodious Conceits* (1573)

6

# THE SEVENTEENTH CENTURY
## The Great Plague, Perfume Fountains and Snuff

These following recipes shall make you walking gardens.

Thomas Jeamson, *Artificiall Embellishments* (1665)

## Introduction

By the beginning of the seventeenth century, the French towns of Grasse and Montpelier were in serious competition with the Italian cities of Venice and Florence when it came to the manufacture and trade of perfume around Europe. Fragrant blooms including carnations, violets, jasmine, roses and lavender were grown in abundance, particularly in the town of Grasse, to satisfy a high demand. The City of London too had become one of the most important trading and business centres in the world. Thomas Gresham's Royal Exchange and New Exchange (effectively early shopping malls) opened in 1570 and 1609 respectively. Both housed countless merchants selling their wares, marking the emergence of shopping as a leisure activity much enjoyed by the aristocracy. Luxury goods from all over the world could be purchased there, including expensive French and Italian perfumes.

Perfumery was an important part of the global economy. The newly established East India Company, which was granted a royal charter in 1600, facilitated the importing of aromatics from the subcontinent into the west to meet the demand for exotic scents. Technological advances in the production of flower waters kept the market buoyant too. Apothecaries argued successfully – under English law, anyway – for the maintenance of their right to sell aromatics as medical treatments. However, selling ready-made perfume was one way for other retail outlets to gain access to this increasingly lucrative business.

While scent continued to be perceived as a prophylactic against illness and a cure for disease it was also quickly becoming something to be enjoyed in its own right. There was an ever-increasing variety of ready-made perfume on the market to choose from if you could afford it. The erotic appeal of perfume was a powerful reason for using it on one's clothes and accessories. Perfumed goods, particularly gloves or jewellery, were must-have possessions for the upper classes.

Floral perfumes were in favour at the beginning of the seventeenth century, but by the second half of the period these had been overtaken again in popularity by stronger-smelling animalic scents such as civet and musk, which were likely to be more effective at covering up any unpleasant odours that might emanate from oneself, other people or one's surroundings. However, there was room for all tastes, and in the seventeenth century a fragrance could be still floral or musky depending on preference.

Although making your own perfume could be cheaper than purchasing a readymade scent, it must be borne in mind that many of the ingredients required to produce the finished fragrance were still very costly so the distinction between purchasing a ready-made perfume and making your own (though the former might be interpreted as a more overt demonstration of wealth and status) was by no means clear cut. Hence, among the wealthier families, aromatics to make luxury scents still ate up a considerable proportion of the household budget. In 1689, the Earl of Bedford 'paid for powder for linen, hair and hands, for the Queen of Hungary's water, for orange water for essence and balls etc a total of two pounds and four shillings'. We don't know what quantities he got for his money, but we might deduce that spending such a large amount of money on the wherewithal to make a perfume explains why some among the aristocracy felt the need to oversee the manufacture themselves. By the seventeenth century, however, it was more usual to employ stillroom maids to do the actual work.

## Perfume in Print

> Thus, as in silver coach she's hurled,
> She both enlightens and perfumes the world.
> Of Aurora Goddess of the Dawn.
>
> Lady Hester Pulter (*c.* 1605–1678)

Scent remained a popular feature of poetry (as in the example above) and didactic works such as housekeeping and cookery books as well as scientific and medical manuals. The proliferation of printed texts furnished a market that was not only interested in purchasing scent but still engaged in making fragrances at home. However, by the latter half of the seventeenth century the topic of scent was no longer confined to a reference, a section or a chapter in works of this type. In this century, we begin to get whole printed books that deal exclusively with the subject. The first of these, published in 1678 in Venice, unsurprisingly, was entitled *Secreti Nobillissimi dell'Arte Profumatoria*, or *The Secret and Most Noble Art of Perfume Making*. Written by the mysterious Giovanventura Rosetti, this work signals the start of a very gradual separation of perfumery and medicinal scent making.

The book was quite quickly followed by two works by the French perfumer Simon Barbe. The first, entitled *Le Parfumeur François* (1693), was aimed at those making their own scent at home and the second, *Le Parfumeur Royal* (1699), was written for any professional businessmen who might work with scent. Barbe himself deemed his second book essential reading for, among others, 'glovers, wigmakers and liqueur sellers'. Even the titles of some of these printed works can give us some insight into the huge range of fragranced goods that could be made up at home or purchased ready for use. Take the title of Barbe's first title when printed in English in 1696: 'The French perfumer teaching the several ways of extracting the odours of drugs and flowers and making all the compositions of perfumes for powder, wash-balls, essences, oyls, wax, pomatum, paste, Queen of Hungary's Rosa Solis, and other sweet waters ...: also how to colour and scent gloves and fans, together with the secret of cleansing tobacco and perfuming it for all sorts of snuff, Spanish, Roman, &c. / done into English from the original printed at Paris.'

The book would no doubt have been valuable reading for those well-to-do ladies who still viewed making perfume as an absorbing hobby. These women too were knowledgeable about the processes of production and included instructions as to how to make perfume in their own family recipe books, not least because of the importance of scent in cookery and medicines (tasks which were the ultimate responsibility of the lady of the house). We find comments on fragrances in their diaries and in private letters too. Cookery writer Lady Anne Fanshawe (1625– 1680), the wife of Sir Richard Fanshawe, the British ambassador to Spain, noted that 'all perfumes are best made in July'. Lady Fanshawe may also have intended to make some considerable amount of the finished product before the raw materials went out of season and therefore build up a supply for the winter. *Queen Elizabeth's Closet of Physical Secrets*, published posthumously in 1656, though in essence a collection of medical prescriptions for plague, smallpox and childbirth complications, also makes reference to perfumes for summer and winter.

## Perfume and Politics

Not only did printed texts preserve the recipes themselves – and by attributing them to notable aristocratic women add prestige to particular formulas – but a few of these books had political purpose and far-reaching implications. One such text was *The Queen's Closet Opened*. The queen referred to in the title is Henrietta Maria (1609–1669), wife of Charles I. Written by one W. M. (possibly Walter Montagu, the eponymous queen's private secretary), the work was published in three sections bound together in 1655. The sections were 'The Pearl of Practice', which dealt with medical remedies; 'A Queen's Delight', concerning confectionery; and 'The Compleat Cook', a collection of general cookery recipes and instructions. The second section was subtitled 'A Right Knowledge of making Perfumes and Distilling the most Excellent Waters'.

The contents throughout are purported to be recipes dear to Henrietta Maria, who at this time was exiled in France while Oliver Cromwell was in charge. The book appealed to popular interest in the lives of royalty; the supposedly personal details of the royals that appear in print today fulfil the same purpose. However, the political influence of the book lay in the fact that it created an image of the exiled queen as housewife and mother. Henrietta Maria had been viewed with suspicion by many of the English aristocracy because she was both Catholic and French. Come the Restoration, the book, which had proved extremely popular (it would run to ten editions), stood her in good stead with the English public. Although she never returned to England for long, Henrietta Maria did visit and had a sizable pension settled on her.

In contrast, a satirical cookery book published at the Restoration was attributed to Elizabeth Cromwell, wife of Oliver Cromwell. This book was intended to show the supposed author as mean and austere despite the fact that Cromwell himself had moved in powerful and wealthy circles where scent was very much seen as a sensory symbol of wealth, status and power. Indeed, he received some beautiful gifts including a Florentine perfume cabinet. Cromwell also personally much favoured scented gloves. In reality, it was unlikely that there was any stinting on luxuries in the Cromwell household.

## Scenting the Environment

One might have said that in the seventeenth century if you ventured outside you did so at your peril. Particularly for those living in the larger European cities, whether France, Italy, Spain or Britain, the smell of their surroundings could be a health hazard. Effluence of all sorts was routinely tipped into rivers. There was a lack of proper drainage and industries gave off all kinds of stench, billowing smoke and dirt. In the seventeenth century the waters of the River Thames were contaminated with human excrement, the bodies of dead animals and the toxic waste from tanning works. Not only was the risk to health significant, but the smell must have been awful.

Given that people at this time still thought of disease as something chiefly transmitted through bad air ('miasma'), counteracting the prevailing stench with the sweet smell of perfume remained very important. Indeed, whether living in the cities, the towns or the countryside the wider populace continued to depend upon scent. In his book *Fumifugium: The Inconvenience of the Aer and Smoak of London Dissipated*, first printed in 1661, John Evelyn suggested a number of measures to purify the air in his city. One of his plans was to plant scented shrubs comprised of 'the most fragrant and odiferous flowers ... aptest to tinge the Aer upon every gentle emission at as great distance'. Privately, in similar vein to the public venture mooted by Evelyn, the wealthy at their country residences grew camomile lawns and constructed knot gardens of scented flowers and herbs such as rosemary, sage and lemon both for enjoyment and to clear the air. Of course they also made practical use of the plants in cookery and medicine as well as making scent.

## Perfumes and the Plague

> Take Angelica roots, and dry them a very little in an Oven, or
> by the fire: and then bruise them very soft, and lay them in Wine
> Vinegar to steep, being close covered three or four days, and then

heat a brick hot, and lay the same there one very morning: this is excellent to air the house or any clothes, or to breath over in the morning fasting.

'Dr Atkinson's Excellent Perfume against the Plague',

*The Queens Closet Opened* (1659)

In 1665, London succumbed to the Great Plague. People looked to pleasant odours just as they had done in the past to protect them and to stem the outbreak of disease. In *The Queens Closet Opened* we find scented cures for the plague among the culinary and other medicinal recipes. These remedies include Dr Atkinson's aromatic cure quoted above. In less complicated fashion, and undoubtedly as a speedier precaution, people tied bunches of lavender to their wrists to ward off the plague. Cinnamon, juniper, cassia and cardamom were burnt both outside in the streets and inside private houses and public buildings in order to dispel the smell of infected bodies and to drive out the disease itself.

Rue, rosemary, cloves, labdanum, cinnamon and other aromatics, as well as exuding a pleasing scent, were all believed effective against plague. The French doctor Philibert Guibert wrote *The Charitable Physician*, a work that was published posthumously (he died in 1633) in English in 1639. Guibert noted, 'Perfumes are certaine medicaments simple and compounded that which without putting in the fire will alter the head and hinder all ill smells and corruption of the aire.' He recommended 'Odiferent candles against venome and the plague', the potential ingredients of which included red roses, cloves, storax, labdanum, benjamin, frankincense, lavender, satinwood, juniper, musk and ambergris. These scented candles were a far cry from the ordinary candles made of tallow, animal fat melted to remove impurities and then hardened.

In physician Thomas Jeamson's *Artificiall Embellishments; or, Art's best Directions how to preserve Beauty or procure it* (1665), the recipes given for perfumes are little more than elaborate versions of contemporary plague remedies. The effectiveness of any of these potential cures probably exists as much in the emotional and physiological effects of their smell as any practical use they might have. Jeamson may have ultimately rued the publication of his book, as he was much ridiculed for it on account of its supposed frivolity. In a chapter on powders for hair, linens and sweet bags Jeamson writes, 'Ladies ... this chapter teaches ye how you shall tickle his nose and fetch him about with a pouder which will give ye so rich a cent that the roses and violets in all your cheeks shall not make you half so sweet.' Although a recognised function of perfume, this was looked down upon by those falling on the medicinal side of scent.

As mentioned previously, when a household suffered an outbreak of illness the residents might resort to calling in a professional fumigator. The windows and doors of the house would be sealed while the fumigator walked from room to room with a hot pan of aromatics. According to the household accounts of Woburn Abbey, the home of the Duke and Duchess of Bedford, following an outbreak of smallpox among the family and their servants in 1641 the duke paid a porter named Antony 5 shillings for pitch and frankincense 'to smoke the house and yard for the purpose of fumigating and disinfecting the house and its environs'. Whether this worked is a matter of conjecture. However, as one might expect, the outbreak of disease certainly had an effect on the price of aromatics. In times of plague the costs simply soared. According to the English playwright Thomas Dekker (*c.* 1572–1632), when the plague was rampant 'rosemary which had wont to be sold for twelve pence an armful was sold for six shillings a handful'.

## The Plague Doctor

Their hats and cloaks of fashion new
are made of oilcloth dark of hue
their caps with glasses are designed
their bills with antidotes all lined.

Anonymous

It is in this century that we first encounter the use of the infamous beaked mask worn by doctors visiting plague victims, widely illustrated and described in contemporary texts. Charles de l'Orme (1584–1678), a physician at the French court in service to no less than three French kings, is credited with inventing the outfit of the plague doctor described in the poem above. It was the hazmat suit of its day. The beak-like nose was of particular importance. Made from either papier-mâché or leather, it was stuffed with sweet-smelling herbs to counteract the actual smell of disease and to give comfort to the medical men. L'Orme himself described the appendage as follows: '[A] nose half a foot long, shaped like a beak, filled with perfume with only two holes, one on each side near the nostrils, but that can suffice to breathe and to carry along with the air one breathes the impression of the drugs enclosed further along in the beak.' Herbs such as camphor, mint, cloves, and myrrh were considered an effective shield for the physician and stored in the beak. On occasion these aromatics were set alight before being put into the beak so that the smoke they gave off might give added protection. While it may have shielded doctors from the smell of death and disease, it probably did little to protect them. As for bedside manner, it can only have been a frightening sight for the plague victim.

## Vinegar of the Four Thieves

There were many who offered perfumed potions to cure disease in the seventeenth century. These fake doctors, originally referred to as quacksalvers, plied their trade across Europe and in the process gave rise to our modern term for an untrustworthy doctor.

Hope seemed on the horizon when a rumour spread that a particularly effective protection against the plague had been found. This perfume became known as the Vinegar of the Four Thieves, and it seems to have originated in the town of Toulouse in France. The inhabitants of the town had been suffering the ravages of an outbreak of the plague from 1628 to 1631, and according to the records of the Parliament of Toulouse, 'during the great plague four robbers were convicted of going to the houses of plague victims strangling them in their beds and them looting their dwellings for this they were condemned to be burned at the stake and in order to have the sentence mitigated they revealed their secret preservative [which allowed them to avoid infection]; after which they were hanged'. The exact context of this story is confused, but the mixture is reputed to have consisted of vinegar heavily laced with garlic and lavender. There is at least a possibility that this might have had some effect; the fact that they did not succumb to plague may have been because the mixture deterred the fleas that were known carriers of the disease. However, modern scholars believe there were other factors that contributed to the spread of the plague (human body lice, for instance), and it is not clear how vinegar would have helped in that case.

## Inside the Home

> Be sure every morning to perfume the house with angelica seeds
> burnt in a fire-pan or chafing dish of coals.
>> M. Stevenson, *The Twelve Months being a treatise*
>> *on Gardening and Husbandry* (1661)

A household of any status did not need the excuse of an outbreak of the plague or some other noxious illness to make copious use of perfume. The mistress of the house was expected to have a knowledge of scent and its applications at her fingertips even if she was not personally engaged in its use or manufacture; if she were wealthy enough such roles would be performed by servants, albeit under her instruction. Perfume cakes might be heated over a fire and used as air fresheners. Floors were still strewn with rushes mixed with herbs like sweet flag, may blossom, lavender or meadowsweet. In poorer homes light came from tallow candles, which did not smell pleasant. The better-off could afford scented candles. In the kitchens the aroma from biscuits and cakes baked using lavender seeds filled the air.

Household manuals still devoted many pages to the topic of scent. In the lengthy title of his book *The English Housewife containing the Inward and Outward Virtues Which Ought to Be in a Complete Woman: as her Phisicke, Cookery, Banqueting-stuffe, Distillation, Perfumes, Wooll, Hemp, Flaxe, Dairies, Brewing, Baking, and all other things belonging to an Houshold* (1615), Gervase Markham (1568–1637) makes sure perfume has its place. The book included a chapter headed 'Of distillations and their virtues and of perfuming', and in it we find stylish and sophisticated recipes for perfume: 'To perfume gloves excellently, take oil of sweet almonds, oil of nutmegs, oil of Benjamin, of each a dram, of ambergris one grain, fat musk two grains: mix them altogether and grind them upon a painter's stone, and then anoint the gloves therewith: yet before you anoint them let them be dampishly moistened with damask rose-water.' Such instructions exist side by side with the mundane work of a country wife.

Away from home, too, the sign of a decent place to stay – 'an honest ale house', as author Izaak Walton (1593–1683) describes it in his *Compleat Angler* – was one where you would 'find a cleanly room, lavender in the windows ... where the linen looks white and smells of lavender'.

## Personal Hygiene

> Others smell so sweetly as if they were new arrived from Arabia
> and brought home perfumes from Horontia.
>
> James Cleland, *The Institution of the
> Young Nobleman* (1607)

In the seventeenth century, hygiene was as important for men as it was for women. Indeed, it remained common practice for both men and women to wash the hands, feet, face and perhaps the intimate parts of their bodies on a regular basis. In his *Laws of Gallantry* (1644), an etiquette book written specifically for male readers, French writer Charles Sorel (1602–1674) stated that 'the whole body should be bathed only occasionally but that a person should wash his hands at least once every day while the face should be washed as often as the hands but the head and hair in most cases only now and then'.

In terms of offering at least the veneer of cleanliness and hygiene, for the wealthy aristocracy, landed gentry and members of the courts of Europe perfume had become an expensive necessity rather than a luxury. Chemist and surgeon John Woodall (1570–1643), in his work *The Surgeons Mate* (1617), recommends formulas 'for the wealthier sort' of 'labdanum ... cloves, cinnamon [and] mirrhe'. For the poorer classes, Woodall suggests a paste made from cloves.

## Fans, Gloves and Aromatic Jewellery

To my Julia lately sent
A bracelet richly redolent
the beads I kissed but most lov'd her
that did perfume the pomander
Robert Herrick (1591–1674)

Perfumed fans were very popular in the seventeenth century. They retained scent well, and when waved about dispensed their fragrance into the air, thus protecting one from the noxious odours about or perhaps even emanating from the person standing or sitting next to you. The fashion for fans would last right up to the mid-nineteenth century. Perfumed gloves held their own as a fashion item too. In France in 1656 the guild of glove and perfume makers was established. This was due to the popularity of perfumed gloves as a fashion that had caught on from Italy in the sixteenth century. John Evelyn refers to 'Gloves trimm'd, and lac'd as fine as Nell [Gwynn]'s. Twelve dozen Martial [presumably a scent named after Martial, the official perfumer of Louis XIV], whole, and half of jonquil, Tuberose, Frangipan, Orange, Violet, Narcissus, Jassemin, Ambrett.'

There was variety of recipes that gave instructions on how to make pomander beads for inclusion in bracelets. From Jeamson's *Artificiall Embellishments* one might try combining 'two ounces of rosebuds the whites being cut off: musk ambergris of each forty grains civet twenty grains: let your roses be beaten fine as usual for conserves then adde the former things with a little labdanum; beat them well together and making them up with gum traganth dissolved in rosewater'. The author promises, in keeping with the tone of his text, that these bracelets on account of their perfume 'will not only bind ... your arms, yet they take men your prisoners'.

Pomanders could still be attached to a chain or worn around the neck rather than incorporated in a bracelet. Small amounts of perfumed gum or powder were also stored in earrings and rings at this time.

## Shopping for Scent

[At] Barnard's Old Perfume Shop (kept by his daughter S Storer)
the sign of the Golden Ball facing the lower end of St James 's
Hay-Market near Pall-Mall London is made and sold all sorts of
perfume wholesale and retail at the lowest prices ...
Handbill for Barnard's Old Perfume Shop (1696)

If you wanted to make your own scent, or even if you wanted to buy a readymade product, where did you go to make your purchase? In the seventeenth century there was plenty of choice. Apothecaries continued to dispense perfumed goods, albeit mostly as treatments for minor ailments such as the lozenges made from musk and aloeswood to treat bad breath. They nonetheless had treatments for trickier problems too, like female infertility; strong scents such as civet, ambergris and musk were to be applied to the female body or burnt in bedchambers when trying to conceive. Specialist perfume shops, meanwhile, sold products in liquid, solid, paste and pastille form. Barbershops also offered scented powder for wigs, which were in style at the time. Household items that doubled as perfume and cooking ingredients could be bought at grocers and other general stockists. Haberdashers sold scented gloves. Royalty might have their own designated suppliers.

## The English Court

When a king (or queen) and their entourage left their dwellings they were of course protected from the unpleasant smells emanating from the inadequate sewers and the thronging crowds. Aside from the individuals themselves carrying scented fans or handkerchiefs, this was done by strewing fragrant flowers and herbs in front of the entourage. In London, mayoral processions too involved scent as an expression of civic and economic power. Spices were thrown into the crowd, perhaps to control the masses but also to protect the great and the good in the procession from the foul smell of the common folk.

By the mid-seventeenth century, the king also employed an official herb strewer whose job it was to mask unpleasant smells in the rooms of the palace by sprinkling fragrant herbs and spices throughout the building as well in front of any royal procession. One Bridget Rumney held this post from 1660 until 1671. She earned £24 a year and a provision of 2 yards of fine scarlet cloth from which to make her uniform. Bridget's employment was interrupted by the Civil War, but following Charles II's return she resumed her position within the court having petitioned the king to allow her to do so. The plants and herbs she used included daisies, fennel, germander, hyssop, lavender, marjoram, maudeline (sweet yarrow), pennyroyal and rose. The last known full-time herb strewer was one Mary Rayner in the eighteenth century. Anne Fellowes, a friend of George IV, would do the job (together with six female attendants) as a one-off on his coronation in 1820.

## The French Court

The French court at Versailles in the reign of Louis XIV became known as *le cour perfume* (the perfumed court), so pervasive was the use of scent by the king and his entourage. There was still a fear of hot water allowing germs in through open pores, so bathing was not part of anyone's regular routine; the French monarch himself is thought to have bathed around three times a year. This surely made for smelly conditions. The palace also had insufficient toilet facilities for the number of residents and visitors, and members of the court were not averse to relieving themselves wherever they felt the need, which would not have helped matters. However, while the smell was due in part to lack of amenities and careless hygiene of the people of the day, no doubt there were also those who did their best within the boundaries of the limited understanding of the time.

Perfume at the French court was not only used to conceal bad odours of course. Its lavish use was also intended to give the impression of luxury, extravagance and sophistication. Notable visitors could expect to be perfumed on their arrival. The reader will not be surprised to know that, just as it had been in the ancient world, the furniture was scented. Bowls of fragrant flowers were strategically placed in all the rooms to counteract foul smells too. Scented fountains were a feature of seventeenth-century dinner parties in fashionable France. These fountains were ornate and luxurious, often made from costly Chinese porcelain, and were therefore in themselves a symbol of the owner's elevated status. These objects were filled with hot scented water which poured forth through spouts made of gilt or bronze to perfume the room.

In his younger days, Louis XIV liked to smell a different fragrance in his rooms every day. However, as he grew older the king seems to have taken a dislike to scent in general, declaring that it made him feel unwell. Nevertheless, he did develop a passion for the scent of orange blossom, establishing an extensive and famous orangery at Versailles. We cannot be sure of the composition of the king's orange blossom scent, but royal perfumer Simon Barbe, in his book *The French Perfumer*, does include the following recipe that dates from the period:

> Orange-flower-water distilled in a cold Still: Infuse two Pounds of Orange-flowers dry in two Pints of Water three or four hours, then pour it in the Still, and distil it as in the former Receipt, the Water distill'd out of it is good for a great many things, as for Wash-balls, to make Angel-water, to cleanse Snuff, and serves to perfume all sorts of Skins and Gloves.

As ever, the love of scent was not confined to the king himself, nor indeed to his womenfolk at court. Clergyman and statesman Cardinal Richelieu (1585–1642), or 'His Red Eminence' as he was known, perfumed his rooms with powder of roses, cypress root, marjoram, cloves, benjamin and storax, all piped through the space by means of bellows. The scent was reputedly so heavy that it made some of his visitors feel sick. It seems that it was not only the French king who found some perfumes and their extravagant use just too much.

## The Affair of the Poisons

Perfume had in the past been implicated in political intrigue, matters of personal jealousy and poisoning, and the seventeenth century was no different. The scandal that became known as The Affair of the Poisons came into being as a result of court gossip between 1677 and 1682 at the French court. Louis XIV's mistress Madame de Montespan was a client of Catherine Monvoisin (1640–1680), known in short as La Voisin, a French fortune teller who dabbled in witchcraft and perfumery. She may or may not have supplied Montespan with a fragrance named *poudre de succession*, a perfumed poison made from arsenic and thallium allegedly intended to eliminate anyone who got in the way of the mistress's pursuit of the king. For her crimes La Voisin in the end met her death by being burnt at the stake for witchcraft, and the deaths laid at her feet are estimated at anywhere between 1,000 and 2,500.

## Famous Perfumes

In the seventeenth century, Hungary water became extremely popular for its scent and its many supposed benefits, which included everything from eternal youth to a cure for gout. One recipe quoted by John Prevot in a medical text published in 1656 was purported to be the original:

> Take of aqua vitae four times distilled three parts and of the tops and flowers of rosemary two parts put these together in a close vessel let them stand in as gentile heat for fifty hours and then distil them take one dram in the morning once every week either in your food or drink and let your face and the diseased limbs be washed with it every morning It renovates the strength brightens the spirits purifies the marrow and nerves restored and preserves the sight and prolongs life.

People drank Hungary water too. According to the day book of an apothecary at the court of William and Mary (dated 1691), one Lord Sussex consumed significant quantities of Hungary water over a period of two years, possibly for toothache or maybe simply as a prophylactic tonic.

Aqua Angeli or angel water was a favourite of Louis XIV of France. He had his shirts rinsed in it. It is thought to have consisted of a mixture of nutmeg, cloves, benzoin, storax and aloeswood. These ingredients needed to be boiled together in rosewater and simmered for around twenty-four hours. After that process was complete, orange flower, jasmine and musk were then added to the reduced pulp.

Citrus-scented neroli or orange flower oil was another popular perfume at this time. Tradition has it that Marie Anne de La Trémoille (1677–1717), princess of the Italian town of Nerola, inspired a fashion for this perfume which she herself had fallen for. In the seventeenth century a technique was developed that allowed this essential oil to be extracted by distillation. The oil extracted from oranges from Seville in Spain was believed to be the best.

Duchess d'Aumont (1650–1711) loved a scent known as Eau à la Maréchale' (or water marshal style) In fact, the perfume was created especially for her in the year 1669. The duchess was the wife of Antoine d'Aumont, Marshal of France and First Gentleman of the Bedchamber. A concoction of iris, nut grass and coriander, Eau à la Maréchale also came in a powdered form for use on hair and wigs known as Poudre à la Maréchale. The duchess is said to have created the hair powder herself.

The scent known as Aqua Mirabilis (miracle water) is believed to have been a precursor to eau de cologne, manufactured in Cologne in Germany from around 1690 by an Italian grocer named Giovanni Pablo Feminis (1660–1736), who had rather mysteriously acquired the recipe from elsewhere. Its light and citrusy scent was in contrast to many of the heavier fragrances that pervaded many private and public spaces. Feminis supposedly added lavender and bergamot to the original mix. The scent was a success, claiming the usual medicinal benefits as well as the pleasure of its scent. The term eau de cologne in later centuries would be used to refer to a light perfume much in keeping with this product.

## Snuff

The taking of snuff – powdered tobacco – had first been observed in the fifteenth century in the Americas by the explorer Christopher Columbus. Its use became popular in France, having been introduced there by Jean Nicot (1530–1600), a French diplomat and scholar who brought the plant from Portugal in the sixteenth century. Although smoking itself was not fashionable in the seventeenth century, the taking of snuff became de rigueur for both men and women. Often it was scented with attar of roses, jasmine or orange oil. While some varieties were named after their place of origin (Havana snuff or Spanish snuff for example), others were named for the perfume that had been added to the basic mixture, like bergamot snuff or orangery snuff. Inhaling this mixture was thought to help maintain good health.

The Prince of Condé (1530–1569), a prominent member of the French court, liked to witness his favourite snuff being scented just as the aristocracy of previous centuries had thought it important to oversee the making of their perfumes. Selling counterfeit goods or substituting a poisonous substance, of course, could have been a relatively simple task and so it was probably wise to keep an eye on things. Sir Kenelm Digby (1603–1665), an adventurer and diplomat with an interest in cookery, wrote a work entitled *The Closet of the eminently learned Sir Kenelm Digby Knight Opened*. In this work he includes perfumes made from damask rose, musk, ambergris and civet that could be used to scent tobacco. Snuff was stocked alongside luxury perfumes. At the end of the seventeenth century, snuff maker and perfumer James Norvock was advertising in the *London Gazette* that he sold 'all sorts of snuffs Spanish and Italian as well as true and large Bologna wash balls and all sorts of rare Spanish perfumes'.

## Miscellaneous Recipes
### Perfumed Paste Beads

Grind the quantity of Amber you please upon a stone of purpose such as the Painters use &c & one quarter part of Algalla [civet]; & the like of Almisile [almizcle or musk] of so much quantity as the Amber & then putt thereunto a little Alquitira [tragacanth gum], & boyle the same together to a Mass, & there of make the Beades with your hands as you please, putting thorough them a thred with a nidle, & so drie them.

Lady Ann Fanshawe, *Letters* (1625–1680)

## Haggis before Robert Burns

Take a calves chaldron [entrails] and parboyle it; when it is cold mince it fine with a pound of beefe suet & penny loafe grated, some Rosemary, tyme, Winter Savory & Penny royall of all a small handful, a little cloves, mace, nutmeg, & Cinamon, a quarter of a pound of currants, a little suger, a little salt, a little Rosewater all these mixt together well with 6 yolkes of Eggs boyle it in a sheepes paunch and so boyle it.

Anonymous, *The Compleat Cook or,*
*The Whole Art of Cookery* (1694)

## A Scottish Hand Water

Put thyme lavender and rosemary confusly together then make a lay of thicke wine lees in the bottom of a stone pot upon which make another aly of the said herbs and then a lay of less and thens oforward lute the pot well bury it in the ground for six weeks distill it a little thereorputb into a basis of common water maketh very sweet washing water.

Rembert Dodoens, *Ram's Little Dodeon* (1606)

## In Praise of Tobacco (a song)

Tobacco's a Physician Good both for Sound and Sickly: T'is a Hot Perfume That expells Cold Rhewme, And makes it flow downe quickly'.

Barten Holyday, *Technogamia* (1618)

## A Pomander against Pestilential Aire

Take labdanum storax of each a dram cloves half a dram camphor, spikenard, nutmeg of each seven grains, beate them into fine powder and make them into bullets with gum dragant dissolved in rose water.

Philibert Guibert, *The Charitable Physician* (1639)

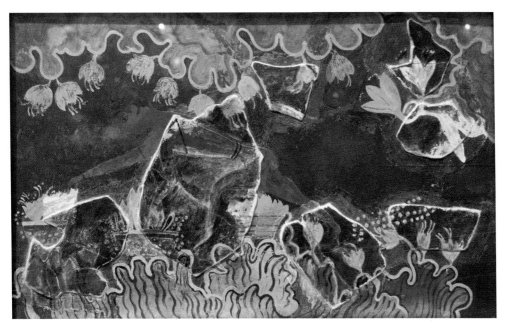

The Blue Boy or Saffron-Gatherer, Minoan fresco from the Palace of Knossos. (Courtesy of Zde under Creative Commons 4.0)

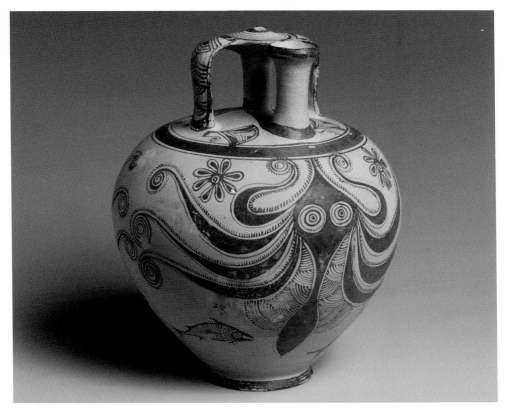

Mycenaean stirrup jar with octopus decoration (1200 BC–1100 BC). (Courtesy of the Metropolitan Museum of Art)

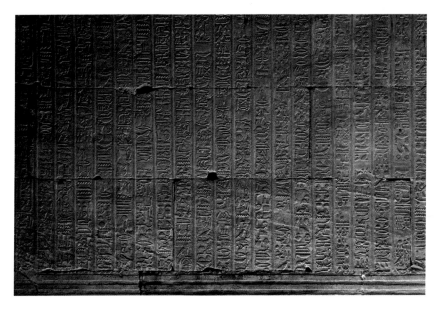

*Above:* Perfume formulas from the Temple of Edfu. (Courtesy of Olaf Tausch under Creative Commons 2.0)

*Below left:* Nefertem depicted with a lotus blossom on his head, based on New Kingdom tomb paintings. (Courtesy of Jeff Dahl under Creative Commons 4.0)

*Below right:* Bronze Etruscan perfume dipper (400 BC–200 BC). (Courtesy of the Metropolitan Museum of Art)

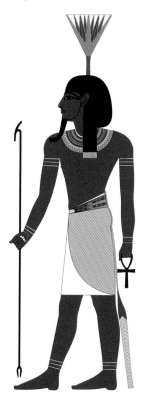

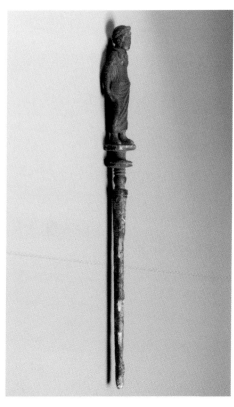

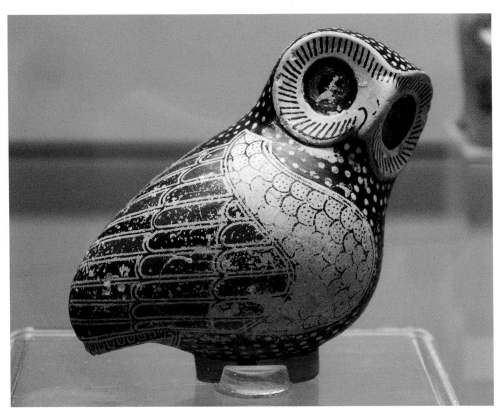

Corinthian *aryballos* in the shape of an owl (*c.* 630 BC). (Courtesy of Carole Raddato under Creative Commons 2.0)

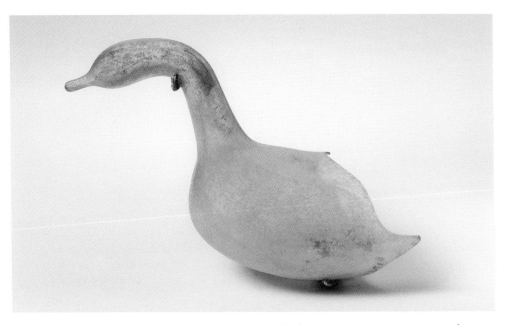

Roman glass perfume bottle in the shape of a bird (1st century AD). (Courtesy of the Metropolitan Museum of Art)

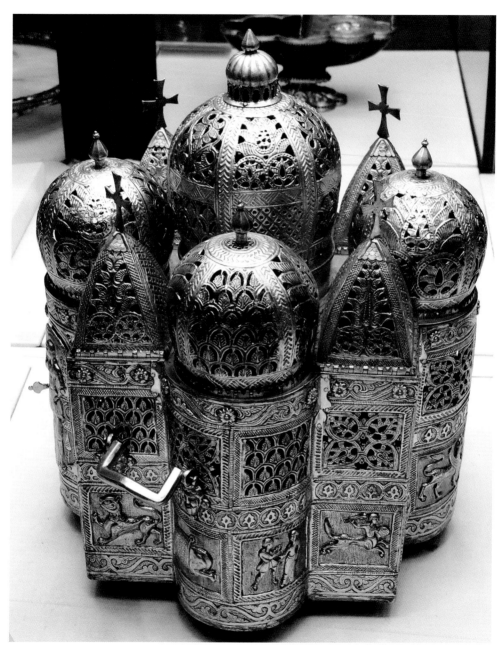

Perfume burner in shape of St Mark's Treasury, Basilica di San Marco, Venice (twelfth century). (Courtesy of Dimitris Kamaras under Creative Commons 2.0)

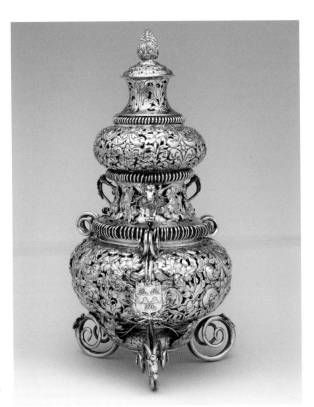

Silver perfume burner
(late seventeenth century).
(Courtesy of the Metropolitan
Museum of Art)

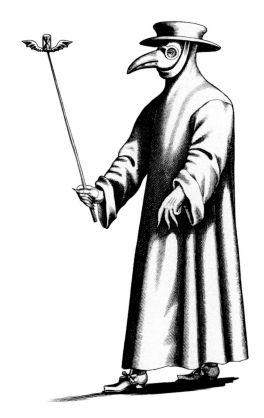

A plague doctor. Based
on Paul Fürst's copper
engraving of Dr Schnabel
from Rome (circa 1656).
(Courtesy of Dv8stees under
Creative Commons 4.0)

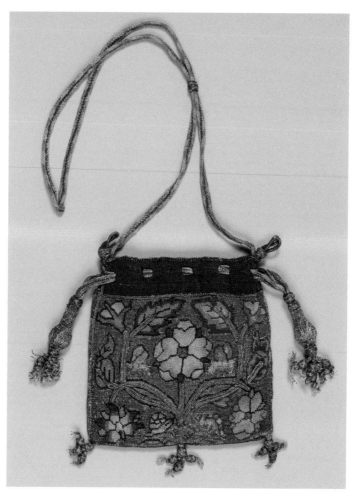

*Above:* Sweet bag (early seventeenth century). (Courtesy of the Metropolitan Museum of Art)

*Below:* Part of the coronation procession of James II (23 April 1685). 'The king's herbswoman and her 6 maids wth baskets of sweet herbs & flowers, strewing the way'. (Courtesy of the Wellcome Library)

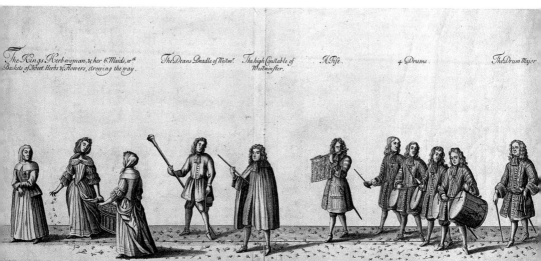

The Kings Herb-woman, & her 6. Maids, wth Baskets of Sweet Herbs & Flowers, strewing the way.    The Deans Beadle of Westmr.    The high Constable of Westminster.    A Fife.    4 Drums.    The Drum Major.

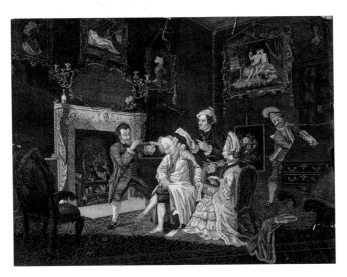

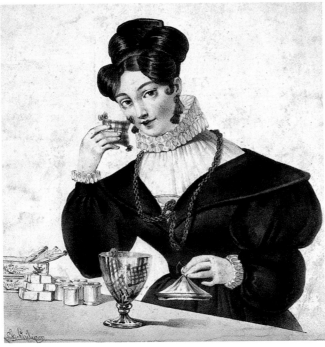

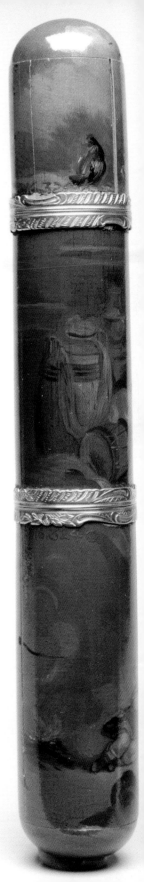

*Top:* Applying scented hair powder, engraving by J. Goldar (1771). (Courtesy of Wellcome Library)

*Above:* Woman perfume seller with a lavender bag (1828), Coloured lithogragh by Charles Philipson.

*Right:* French *etui*, perfume case (*c.* 1780). (Courtesy of Cleveland Museum of Art)

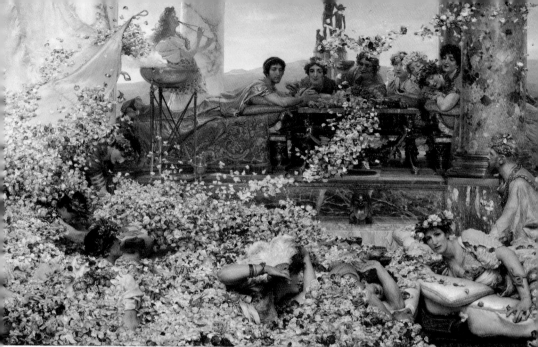

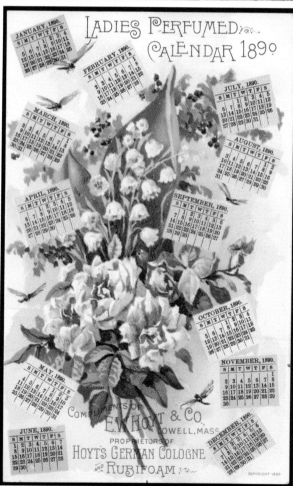

*Above: The Roses of Heliogabalus*, Lawrence Alma-Tadema (1888).

*Left:* Perfumed calendar, (1890). (Courtesy of Boston Public Library)

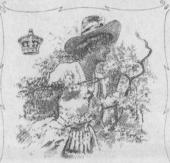
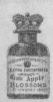
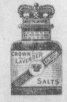
Trade card for the Crown Perfumery Company (nineteenth century). (Courtesy of Boston Public Library)

Trade card for Atkinsons perfume (nineteenth century). (Courtesy of Boston Public Library)

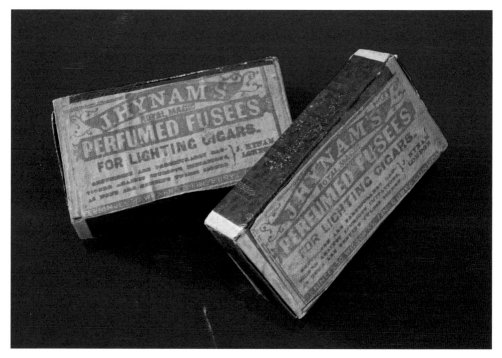

Two boxes of J. Hynam's perfumed fusee matches. (Courtesy of the Wellcome Library)

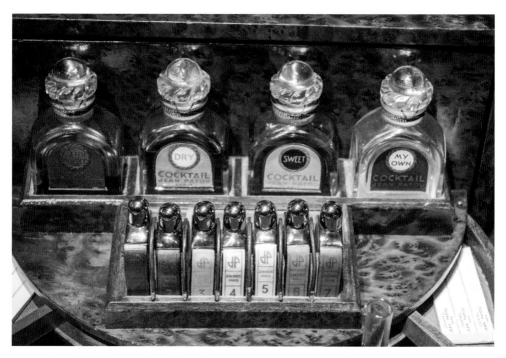

A cocktail bar perfume box by Jean Patou. (Courtesy of Tim Evenson under Creative Commons 2.0)

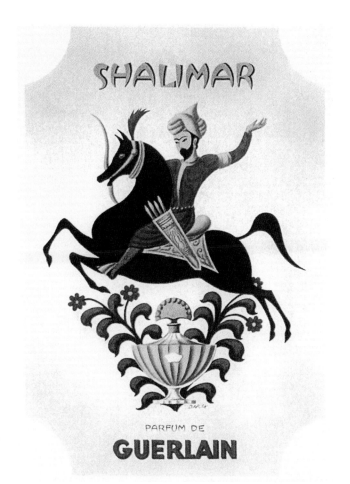

Advertisment for
Shalimar by Guerlain.
(Courtesy of Darcy
Lyse under Creative
Commons 1.0)

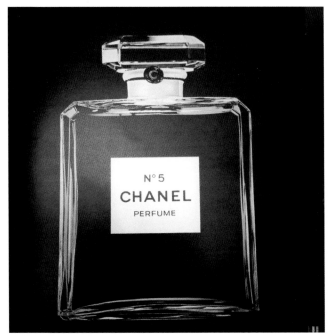

Chanel No. 5.
(Courtesy of Romana
Klee under Creative
Commons 2.0)

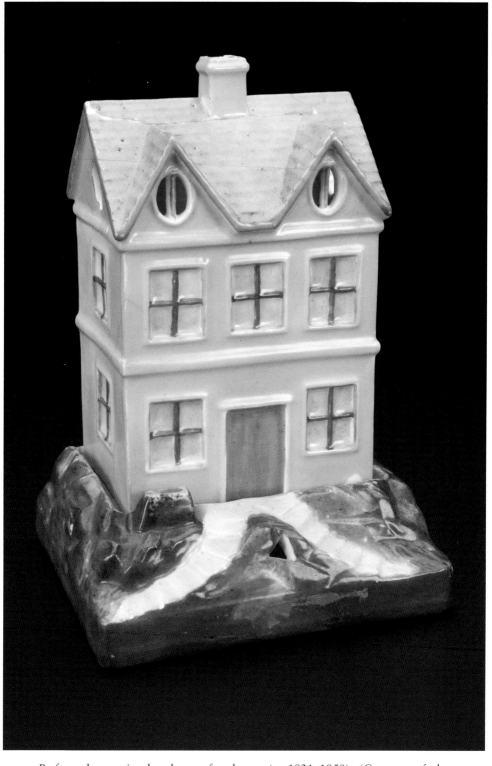

Perfume burner in the shape of a house (*c*. 1821–1850). (Courtesy of the Wellcome Library)

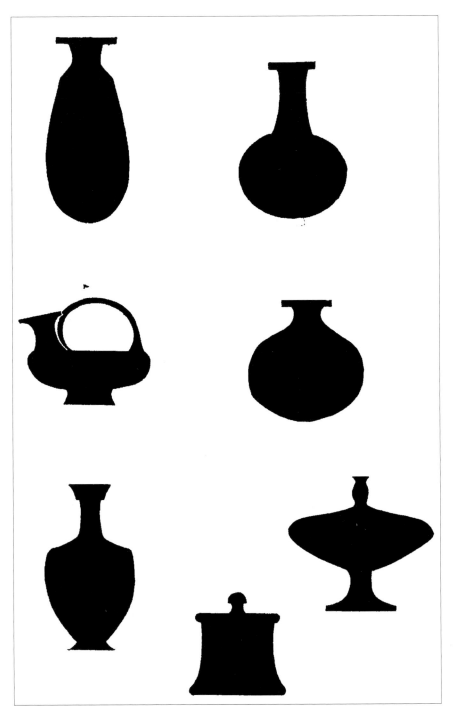

Bottle shapes from top left clockwise: alabastron, ampulla, aryballos, exleiptron, pyxis, lekythos, askos. (By kind permission of artist Chris Sutherland)

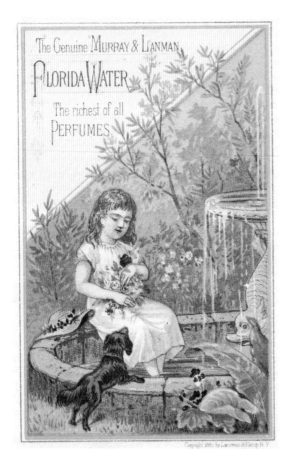

*Left:* An advertisement for Florida Water. (Courtesy of Boston Public Library under Creative Commons 2.0)

*Below:* Nip sampling container. Nips was a patented name for a method of perfume sampling from the 1930 to 1950s. (Courtesy of LBCC Historical Apothecary)

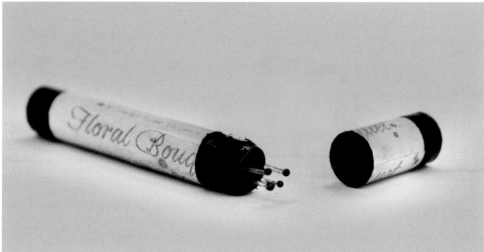

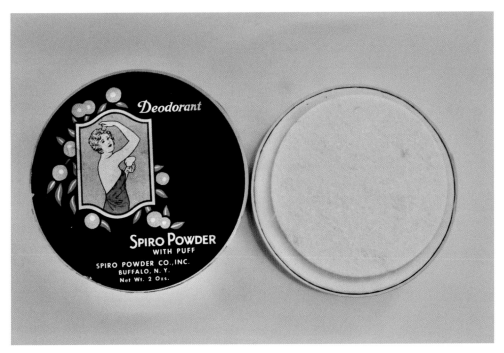

BUY
*Indian Queen Perfume*
AND HAVE
**PERFUMED CARDS**
PRINTED WITH YOUR NAME AND BUSINESS ON.

**BEAN & RABE,**
**PROPRIETORS,**
*47 & 49 NORTH SECOND STREET,*
Philadelphia.

Indian Queen Perfume promotional material. (Courtesy of Boston Public Library under Creative Commons 2.0)

Spiro Deodorant Powder, early 1930s. (Courtesy of LBCC Historical Apothecary)

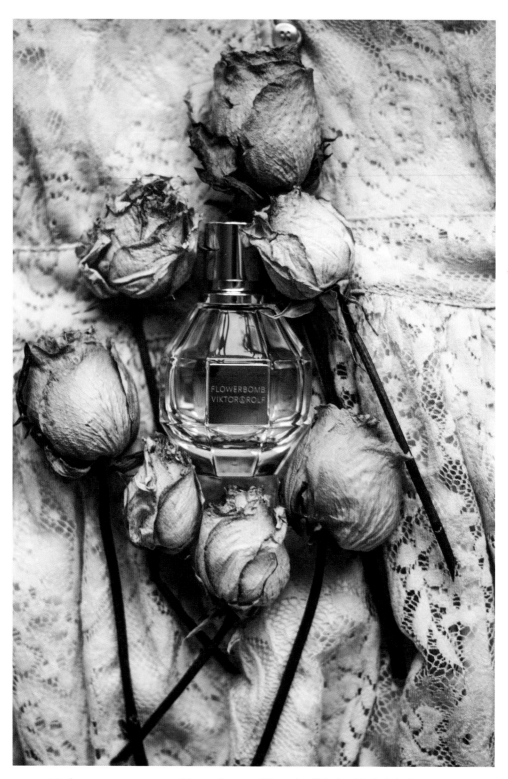

Modern scent – our eternal love of roses. (Photo by Kristina Paukshtite)

## Damask Rose Syrup

Pour boiling water on a quantity of damask roses just enough to cover them. Let them stand four and twenty hours then press off the liquor and add to it twice the quantity of sugar. Melt this and the syrup is completed.

Thomas Tryon, *A Treatise of Cleanness in Meates* (1682)

## Rose Sugar Mix

Take fresh red Roses not quite ripe, beat them in a stone Mortar, mix them with double their weight of Sugar, and put them in a glass close stopped, being not full, let them remain before you use them three moneths, stirring of them once a day. The Vertue. The Stomach, Heart, and Bowels it cooleth, and hindereth vapours, the spiting of blood and corruption for the most part (being cold) it helpeth. It will keep many years.

Anonymous, *The Queen's Closet Opened* (1655)

## Conserves of Violets in the the Italian Manner

Take the leaves of blew [blue] violets separated
from their stalks and greens beat
them very well in a stone mortar with
twice the weight of sugar and reserve
them for your use in a glass vessel.

Anonymous, *The Queen's Closet Opened* (1655)

## A Winter Scent

Red-Roses Marjoram and Myrtles, of either a little handful: Callamint, Juniper berries, Labdanum, Benjamin, and Frankincense, of either {dram}. i. which is the weight of seven pence. The hearbs, berries, and Roses being dried, must be made in grosse powder, as also the gumms, and so mixed together, and when yee list, cast some part there of on a chafer of coales, and receive the fume thereof.

Anonymous, *The Queen's Closet Opened* (1655)

## To Perfume Water

Take Malmsey or any kinde of sweet
water, then take Lavander, Spike, sweet
Marjoram, Balm, Orange peels, Thime,
Basil, Cloves, Bay leaves, Woodbine
flowers, red and white Roses, and still them all together.

Anonymous, *The Queen's Closet Opened* (1655)

## Rose Pastils to Burn

Take Benjamin three ounces storax two ounces. Alexandrine or damask rose buds one ounce: grind the roses by themselves and the rest also: Then take lignum aloes amber fine sugar civet powder of cypress of each half a quarter of pounds. Grind all these well together. Then mix with gum tragacanth in orange flower or rosewater to make them up.

Sir Kenelm Digby, *The Closet of the
Eminently Learned Sir Kenelm Digby
Knight Opened* (1669)

## A Bag to Smell unto for Melancholy or to Cause One to Sleep

Take drie rose leaves keep them close in a glasse which will keep them sweet then take powder of mints powder of clove in a grosse powder and put the same to the rose leaves then put all these together in a bag and take that to bed with you and it will cause you to sleep and it is good to smell unto at other times.

Rembert Dodoens, *Ram's Little Dodeon* (1606)

## To Scent a Candle

Take Benjamin storax oz each foure oz. frankincense olibanum or each 12oz. labdanum 18 oz nigela 1 oz coriander seeds juniper berries of each halfe an oz, liquid storax sixe oz turpentine half an oz. form this into candles with gum dragant and rosewater.

Philibert Guibert, *The Charitable Physician* (1639)

## A Pleasant and Wholesome Perfume for Tobacco Taken in a Pipe

Take one ounces of hard balsom that is in nuts ambergris half a dram oyl of aniseeds six drops oyl of cinnamon six or seven or ten drops oyl of thyme five drops oyl of nutmeg, oyl of lavender of each two drops oyl of cloves three drops work all these together by long malaxations in a mortar warmed a little into an uniform gummy substance whereof as much as a peppercorn pressed in at the top of a pipe of tobacco will make it taste exceedingly well and perfume the mouth and room very pleasantly by taking it in smoke'

Kenelm Digby, *The Closet of the Eminently Learned Sir Kenelm Digby Knight Opened* (1669)

## A Good Perfume in Summer Season

Conserve of the flowers of lavender Take the flowers being new so many as you pleases and beat them with three times their weight of white sugar after the same manner as rosemary flowers; they will keep for one year

Anonymous, *The Queen's Closet Opened* (1655)

Note: According to Hugh Platt's *Delights for Ladies*, rosemary flowers needed to be 'pounded in a stone mortar' then put into 'well glazed gallipots'.

## Another Good Perfume in Summer Season

Rx. Rose water and Vinegar, of either six spoonfuls: Rinds of sower Citrons and Lemons, Bay-leaves, of either the weight of two pence which is i. Camphire, the weight of three pence, which is 3. ss. The hearbs and rinds must be dried and put alltogether in a perfuming pan, or instead thereof a peuter dish, set on a chafer of coles, will serve the turn.

Anonymous, The Queen's Closet Opened (1655)

## King Edward the Sixths Perfume

Take twelve spoonfuls of right red rosewater the weight of six pence in fine powder of sugar and boyl it on hot embers and coals softly and the house will as though it were full of roses but you must burn the sweet cypress wood before to take away the gross ayre.

Anonymous, The Queen's Closet Opened (1655)

## To Scent Tobacco

Take Balm of Peru half an ounce, seven or eight Drops of Oyl of Cinnamon, Oyl of Cloves five drops, Oyl of Nutmegs, of Thyme, of Lavender, of Fennel, of Aniseeds (all drawn by distillation) of each a like quantity, or more or less as you like the Odour, and would have it strongest; incorporate with these half a dram of Ambergris; make all these into a Paste; which keep in a Box; when you have fill'd your Pipe of Tobacco, put upon it about the bigness of a Pin's Head of this Composition. It will make the Smoak most pleasantly odoriferous, both to the Takers, and to them that come into the Room; and ones Breath will be sweet all the day after. It also comforts the Head and Brains. Approved by Sir Kenelm Digby.

George Hartman, The True Preserver and<br>Restorer of Health (1682)

## An Excellent Odoriferous Perfume for Chambers and Rooms of Entertainment, Much Used in France

Take the powder of Willow coals three ounces, Labdanum two ounces, Store and Benja|min, of each half an ounce, Mastick, sweet Taccamahacca, and yellow Amber, of each two drams; Lignum Rhodium a dram and half; re|duce them all into a subtil Powder, and make them up into small Candles with Gum Tragant steep'd in Rosewater, then dry them in the sha|dow; kindle the narrow end of them, and set them in a Candlestick, or heat the Pin of a Save-all, and then thrust it into the bigger end and so set it upon a Candle-stick.

George Hartman, *The True Preserver and Restorer of Health* (1682)

## A Delicate Washing Ball

Take three ounces of orace halfe an ounce of cypre two ounces of calamus aromaticus one ounce of rose leaves two ounces of lavender flowers beat all these together on a mortar searcing then through a fine search.

Sir Hugh Platt, *Delights for Ladies* (1656)

## A Famous Odoriferous Sweet Water Call'd the Angel's Water

Take Roots of Florence Orrice and Benjamin, of each an ounce and half, select Storax six drams, Lignum Rhodium half an ounce, Aromatic Reed, and Labdanum, of each two scruples, Flowers of Benjamin a scruple; pulverize them all, and put them into a Mattress, or in a strong Bottle, and pour upon it a pint of Rose-water, and half a pint of Orange-flower-water; Stop the Bottle or Mattress very close, and set it in lukewarm water for twenty four hours; then distil in a Cucurbite in Balneo Mariae, and keep the water for Use: If you please you may mix it with Musk and

Ambergris; or you may put in it a few drops of the Essence of Amber, afterwards set down.

This Water is call'd The Angels-Water, be|cause of its sweet and pleasing Odour; you may, after you have infused the Ingredients in the Waters, strain the Infusion, and having dissolv'd in it the Musk and Ambergrease, keep the Li|quor for Use, without distilling it. Of the Se|diments you may make sweet Bags to put a|mong Cloaths and Linnen.

Sir Hugh Platt, *Delights for Ladies* (1656)

## Air Freshener Known as the Perfume of King Henry the Eighth

Of compound water [aqua composita'] six spoonfuls, as much of rose-water, a quarter of an ounce of fine sugar, two grains of musk, two grains of amber-grease, two of civet: boyl it softly together: all the housewill smell of cloves.'

Sir Hugh Platt, *A Closet for Ladies* (1618)

Note: As an alterative, and also according to Sir Hugh Platt, Edward VI's perfume would 'make your house smell of rosemary'.

## Perfume to Wear about You

Beat in a little mortar the bigness of a pea of Benjamin pir over it a few drops of Balm of Peru: then add to it four grains of civet stir it and mix it well with the pestle and put it with cotton in your perfume box.

Simon Barbe, *The French Perfumer* (1696)

# 7

# THE EIGHTEENTH CENTURY
## Macaronis, Spas and Perfume Houses

And first a dirty smock appeared,
Beneath the armpits well besmeared.
Strephon, the rogue, displayed it wide,
And turned it round on every side.
On such a point few words are best,
And Strephon bids us guess the rest,
But swears how damnably the men lie,
In calling Celia sweet and cleanly.

Jonathan Swift, 'The Lady's
Dressing Room' (1732)

## Introduction

Poet and cleric Jonathan Swift (1667–1745), most famous for his novel *Gulliver's Travels*, makes much of bad smells in his scatological poem 'The Lady's Dressing Room', from which the above quotation is taken. His accusations of bad odour, which he makes elsewhere as well as in this example, were generally directed at women; Swift had a reputation as a misogynist. Though no doubt the extent of the prevailing bad odour has been exaggerated, it is true to say that in the eighteenth century unpleasant smells remained a reality. Waste from private homes and commercial premises, poor personal hygiene (certainly by modern standards), horse excrement in the streets, crowded city living conditions and a lack of knowledge about food preservation were just a few of the things that combined to produce pervasive and noxious smells at this time.

Paris and London were by now Europe's largest cities, and the French dramatist Louis-Sébastien Mercier (1740–1814) is on record declaring that Paris, as well as being one of the largest cities, was also *the* 'dirtiest city in the world': 'One must walk through a liquid muck black and stinking and reaching to one's calf.' Little wonder, then, that people persisted in using perfume to fragrance the air and themselves as well as their homes and their belongings. Indeed, the popularity of scent hardly wavered throughout the eighteenth century, and would survive even the turmoil and upheaval caused by the French Revolution beginning in 1789.

During the course of the eighteenth century there was some progress made in perfume production methods, including an improvement in distillation techniques which allowed for faster and somewhat cheaper manufacture. However, enfleurage (the immersion of aromatics in a warm fat which captures their scent) was still being used for the most fragile of plants, including the ever-popular rose and jasmine. Enfleurage was a slow and laborious process which kept the prices of the increasingly fashionable florals beyond the reach of the general public.

As to the long-established association of scent with medicine, while this may have drifted a little by the eighteenth century it was very much alive. Chemists sold perfumes as well as remedies and a sweet odour was still seen as a powerful component of any medical cure. Aromatics, such as musk and amber, sought after for their scent, were also used to treat coughs and colds. The virtues of a pleasant odour remained a theme in religious contexts too. The Catholic, High Anglican and Greek Orthodox churches continued to burn incense as part of their worship, particularly frankincense and myrrh. Scent was still an indication of sainthood. In 1757 the German archaeologist and travel writer J. G. Keyssler (1693–1743) noted that 'St. Antony's remains [in Padua] is said continually to emit a most fragrant perfume', though he does not claim to have observed this miracle himself.

## Animal Excreta and Floral Scent

> However disgusting as all animal perfumes must be there has been a time when the produce of the civet's posterior was in the highest esteem with the ladies and effeminate men ... the very idea of borrowing from such a source is not a little offensive to a delicate mind. The traffic in this perfume however is still very considerable ... but to the credit of taste and elegance it is now greatly on the decline.
>
> William Fordyce Mavor, *Natural History for the Use of School* (1800)

Animal excreta – specifically musk, civet, ambergris and castoreum (beaver oil) – remained fashionable with many people in the eighteenth century, if for no other reason than their strength meant they stood a better chance of covering up the most noxious of odours that one could encounter on a daily basis. Aside from the need to cover up bad smells and follow fashions, a lady's or gentleman's choice of scent was also a matter of personal preference and some of these heavy scents did not appeal to everyone. In the first year of the century, English sugar merchant Thomas Tyron (1634–1703) remarked, in a letter headed 'The Nature of Smells', that musk 'was the dearest of Stinks: and if Hog's Dung was as scarce, it is probable it might be as much in esteem'. The East India Company banned the transportation of musk on their tea clippers because when the tea arrived at its destination it smelled of musk, affecting the quality and saleability of the cargo. By the end of the century, Scottish educationalist William Fordyce Mavor (1758–1837) could categorically deny the virtues of animal waste (civet in particular) to his audience of school pupils.

Over the century there was, in fact, a slow decline in appreciation for musky scents. Indeed, the eighteenth century generally heralded a trend towards the use of more delicate floral perfumes comprising the essence of one particular flower or herb mixed with alcohol. Rose, lavender, violet, cloves, nutmeg, oakmoss and orris root were all popular. This fashion indicated the growing refinement of the period, suggesting as it does that scents were starting to gain appreciation for their own smell rather than their potency for covering up other, worse smells. In his work *The Toilet of Flora*, Pierre-Joseph Buc'hoz (1731–1807), a French physician whose interest lay primarily in alternative therapies, makes clear his interest in perfume in its own right. Note his comments in the following recipe for a toilette water:

> Take honey-water an ounce eau sans pareille, two ounces jasmine water, not quite five drachms clove water and violet water of each half an ounce, Cyprus water, sweet calamus water and lavender water of each two drachms, spirit of neroli or oranges ten drops mix all the waters together and keep the mixture in a vial corked ... This water has a delightful scent but its use is only for the toilet.

## Newspapers, Broadsides and Trade Cards: The Power of Advertising

While medical books, recipe collections, private inventories and documents both formal and informal continue to be a mine of information on the topic of scent for historians, in the eighteenth century further details can be found in a new range of sources. These include trade cards, broadsheets or handbills, as well as advertisements in newspapers and in a newly emerging range of magazines.

The advertisements for perfume that began to appear in newspapers and magazines followed a fairly standard format. In general they consist of the name and location of the seller together with a list of their products. If the seller could afford it there was an illustration, perhaps indicating royal connections through a motif like the Prince of Wales's feathers. The image of the civet cat, despite the waning popularity of its derivative perfume, appears regularly in eighteenth-century perfume advertisements too. This was sometimes an indication that there was actually a live civet cat on the premises, which was not an uncommon attraction for customers.

The same advertising format that appeared in contemporary newspapers and magazines was used in what were known as broadsides. These were single paper bills or posters that promoted goods for sale. Trade cards too were distributed by retailers and tradesmen to potential customers and gave much the same information as the advertisements that appeared in the other formats, though generally in a more decorative style with a handsome pictorial engraving and copperplate script.

Advertising could showcase the wide range of goods that a particular establishment might have for sale, from scented snuff and expensive French perfumes to wash balls, fragrant hair powders and everyday toilet waters. Advertisements might also promote specifics. In 1708 editions of the British daily newspaper *The Daily Courant* the reader might be enticed by the Princely Perfume, 'a most delightful Powder, which incomparably scents Handkerchiefs, Gloves, and all Sorts of Linnen'. The information given in a newspaper, on a trade card or a broadside often noted that the aforesaid goods were available 'wholesale and retail'.

From these various forms of promotion we learn the names of some of the contemporary fragrances on sale, including Eau de Carmes and Eau sans Pareil. However there is often little or no indication of their ingredients. In the case of others such as Eau de Lys, water perfumed with orris root, and jessamy powder, a hair powder scented with jasmine, we do get more of a sense of their fragrance. The names of these fragrances are often French, but this may be the mere illusion of luxury and prestige rather an indication that the scents were genuinely manufactured in France. Similarly, making a royal connection in the name such as royal water or king's honey water clearly added prestige too.

## *Shopping for Scent*

The eighteenth century saw a significant increase in the production of commercial perfumes manufactured outside the home. Indeed, there was a veritable explosion of readymade scents. According to a 1747 edition of the daily London newspaper *The General Advertiser*, 'At the Italian warehouse the crown in Panton Street near Leicester fields is lately imported the following perfumed waters ... Cyprus pink, jessamean, mistereuse, milfleur martecale, cedrate, bergamot, voilette supreme sans pareil ... French lavender, quintessence of roses, jessamin, pink citron.' The variety of scents on the market seems almost overwhelming.

The number of specialist perfume companies (or 'perfume houses') that sprang up at this time is another indication of the popularity of scent and the variety of readymade products on sale. Perfumers like Charles Lillie, who opened his own shop in The Strand in London as early as 1708 selling 'snuffs and perfumes that refresh the brain', regularly advertised in newspapers and magazines, especially favouring *The Tatler* and *The Spectator*. Lillie was also at the forefront of perfuming snuff and offered demonstrations at his shop for other businesses on how to do this. He also poured scorn on homemade product in his adverts. Whereas country houses and estates of the rich had previously produced their own perfume, those with wealth and a social position to uphold now sought to buy expensive perfumes and other scented goods, especially from France. Another form of advertising also saw its beginnings in the eighteenth century, albeit towards the end of the period. This new means of promotion took the form of small sample bottles, sometimes referred to as 'throwaways'. These bottles were in fact glass tubes hand painted and decorated with gilt and enamel. Perfume sellers handed out these small vials to their clientele to tempt them to buy the full-size product. It seems that the use of the sample as a marketing tool has a longer history than one might imagine.

There was plenty of commercial competition as all sorts of shops made it their business to sell scent; after all, it had long been a lucrative business. The extensive list of retailers who sold such goods still included apothecaries or chemists who had traditionally sold the ingredients to make perfume as well as the new specialist perfume shops set up by the perfume companies themselves. In every town and city there were markets and itinerant street sellers who sold (among other things) wash balls and toilet waters as well as fresh flowers for nosegays. In a story from a children's story book dating from 1797, twin sisters set off to buy themselves nosegays:

> Fanny and Sophia were again invited to the house of a lady, whom, as Fanny regarded her as a person of great taste, she was desirous to please her by appearance. She put on all her little finery, but found that one thing was necessary to complete her dress, which was a nosegay, and this she was determined to buy when they reached the town.

Perfumed goods could also be purchased in clothes shops, milliners, even toyshops and libraries. Mary Sellen, a milliner in Pierpoint Street in Bath, sold fragrant powders and Hungary water alongside her hats. A Mr Whalley of Macclesfield, according to his newspaper advertisement, offered his customers an astonishing range of goods from children's toys to scented French and English powder. In 1784, at Moore's Universal Toy Shop in Bath, 'For Ready Money only ... as well as pocket-books, boxes, gold-pins, lockets, bracelets, trinkets, ear-rings, tooth-pick cases, purses, Paris irons, combs that will not split ... one might purchase perfumery of this year's growth, from abroad, rose pomatum at 1s. per pot ... gentlemen's silk bags ... hair powder of better quality than any yet sold.' The library manual *The Use of Circulating Libraries Considered* (1797) maintained that 'not one Circulating Library in twenty' could make any money unless it combined book borrowing with another business. Selling perfumes was one option.

## Making Your Own

The making of one's own scent at home continued in the face of commercial competition. Despite the plethora of readymade perfume on sale the gardens of many grand houses and estates could, and did, provide the necessary floral and herbal needs of the household when required. There were plenty of books that continued to address the private individual or amateur perfume maker rather than the professional.

Aside from the availability of the ingredients in one's own garden, cutting the cost was a factor in making your own scented goods whether liquid, solid, perfumed waters, hair powders, soaps or lotions. While readymade perfumes could be bought quite easily, they did come at a price. However, the more exotic ingredients that someone might want to purchase to make their own fragrance at home could also be expensive. Take civet for example. Used for its own smell and as a fixative for other scents, it held its value despite a steady decline in interest. This may have been because even in the middle of the eighteenth century civet was still seen as a panacea as well as a way of scenting the linen. According to *The Ladies Dispensatory or Every Woman her Own Physician*, published around 1755, ten grains of civet cost 2 shillings, ten times the price of a hot meal or enough coal to last the day. Such exotic ingredients were not within the grasp of the poor.

Another problem that dogged the perfume industry was the fact that the high cost in making some perfumes tempted manufacturers to sell counterfeit goods; fraud is nothing new. Those who made their own could perhaps be surer of the authenticity of the finished product, though they still had to ensure that the ingredients they purchased had not been adulterated.

Writers like Simon Barbe in his manual *The French Perfumer* encouraged those who could not afford to purchase the expensive perfumes (or the more exclusive ingredients) to continue to make their own with what they could. In this way, Barbe stated that his text 'served the publick good'. However, he acknowledged that those wishing to make their own scent needed 'leisure enough to gather the flowers at ... country seats'. His advice could hardly apply to the poorest in that case. Nevertheless, there were those who could 'save the expense of buying those [perfumes] at extravagant rates in shops'.

## Men and Macaronis

> When his Eyes are set to a languishing Air, his Motions all prepar'd according to Art, his Wig and his Coat abundantly Powder'd, his Handkerchief Perfum'd, and all the rest of his Beauty rightly adjusted ... 'tis time to launch, and down he comes, scented like a Perfumer's Shop, and looks like a Vessel with all her Rigging without Ballast.
>
> Abel Boyer, *The English Theophrastus, or Manners of the Age* (1702)

As time went on there were more and more opportunities for men to use perfume, partly due to the contemporary fashion for a clean-shaven face. Shaving soap and scented products for aftercare were advertised in the newspapers and could be purchased for home use or applied at the barbers. Paris pearl water and Persian soap were two possible options believed to soothe the skin after shaving.

The quotation above from Abel Boyer (1667-1729), who once brawled with the aforementioned Jonathan Swift, paints a picture of a gentleman whom we might describe as a Macaroni, the precursor of the nineteenth-century dandy. While accurate, however, his text is slightly too early; in fact, the term Macaroni arrived with the establishment of the Macaroni Club in London in the 1760s by a few wealthy young Englishmen who had just returned from a trip to Italy. According to an anonymous letter published in the London paper *The Weekly Amusement* in 1775, the club was open to new members:

> Macaronis and who can evince that they are men and gentlemen philosophers by explaining to the satisfaction of the original

members of the society the essence of pomatums and puffs and the suction and ebullition of powder bellows.

What is relevant here is the Macaroni's love for, and excessive use of, perfume, above and beyond typical masculine usage at this time. Not only did a Macaroni heavily perfume his wig, his clothes and his accessories (his handkerchief, for example) but he might carry a small nosegay as he went about town much in the fashion of women of the day. The word jessamy (an old word for jasmine) came to refer to a dandy as these foppish young men liked to wear a sprig of jasmine as a buttonhole.

For their devotion to scent and their flamboyant dress the Macaronis were frequently criticised and their sexuality was called into question. However, others wrote in support of fragrance. Among them were those whose fascination seems to have been inspired by their interest in gardening. Poet and landscape gardener William Shenstone (1714–1763) expressed a view contrary to the disparaging opinions expressed about scent; note his subject is male although that may be generic.

> Why are perfumes so much decryed? When a person, on his approach, diffuses them, does he not revive the idea which the ancients ever entertained concerning the scent of superior beings, 'veiled in a cloud of fragrance'?

We can be sure that for the Macaroni, perfuming oneself was both laborious and expensive. According to a 1743 edition of *The Female Spectator*, an upmarket magazine for women and the more foppish of men, the Macaroni's taste typically required 30 pounds of perfumed powder (costing £1 1s), six pounds of jessamine butter for one's hair (at the princely sum of £6 6s) and six bottles of orange flower water (at the even more exorbitant price of £11) as well as a quantity of bergamot snuff and perfumed mouth water.

## Powdered Wigs

The popularity of powdered wigs also encouraged the use of perfume by both sexes. Popular perfumes for powders included jasmine, rose, hyacinth, narcissus (daffodil) and orange blossom. The chosen scent was mixed with starch and ground bones to make the finished product. Both men and women wore these wigs perfumed with powder and kept in shape by sticky, scented pomades traditionally based on bear's fat. In 1791, botanist Mary Frampton (1773–1846) noted in her diary:

> The ladies wore the hair flowing down their backs and high in front, with much pomatum and powder put on with different kinds of puffs. The finishing powder had a brown hue and a strong perfumed smell, and was called 'Maréchale' powder. This powder was applied at a distance, that every hair might be frosted with it. One pound, and even two pounds, of powder were sometimes put into the hair or wasted in the room in one dressing.

Applying hair powder was certainly a messy business, often carried out in an anteroom using a paper cone to direct as much of the powder onto the hair as possible. The popularity of the powdered wig endured until a little before the end of the eighteenth century.

## Scent and Sickness: The French Pox and Smallpox

The health benefits of fragrance remained significant to both medical professionals and the wider public, with the latter clinging to the idea that perfume, in the absence of much else, was a prophylactic and a cure. The idea that you called upon a perfumer to fumigate your house after an outbreak of illness held, at least for the first part of the century. There were health benefits to be had from adding scent to food and drink, too, as in this quote from French dramatist Louis-Sébastien Mercier:

> The dishes of the present day are very light, and they have a particular delicacy and perfume. The secret has been discovered

of enabling us to eat more and to eat better, as also to digest more rapidly ... The new cookery is conductive to health, to good temper, and to long life.

In 1777, Pierre Lalouette (1711–1792), a renowned French anatomist, invented a fumigation machine that dispensed perfume as a cure for syphilis or 'French pox', which was a serious problem at the time. The ingredients dispensed by Lalouette's invention included frankincense, nutmeg, myrrh, juniper, mercury and sulphur – an abrasive and caustic mixture which probably did more harm than good. For another serious disease prevalent in the eighteenth century, smallpox, Lady Catherine Stewart recommended alum boiled in milk 'to hinder the smallpox from pitting by stroaking the pustules as they come out'. Lady Stewart also suggested a mixture of fragrant plant material in this prescription, using General Wade's Admirable Balsam, which contained 'Balsam Peru, storax Calamis, St. Johns Wort flowers. Benjamine, Sweet Almonds, Frankincense, Angelica roots, all infused in spirit of wine'.

## Aromatic Baths and Spa Delights

Boil, for the space of two or three minutes, in a sufficient quantity of river-water, one or more of the following plants; viz. Laurel, Thyme, Rosemary, Wild Thyme, Sweet-Marjoram, Bastard-Marjoram, Lavender, Southernwood, Wormwood, Sage, Pennyroyal, Sweet-Basil Balm, Wild Mint, Hyssop, Clove-July-flowers, Anise, Fennel ... have an agreeable scent. Having strained off the liquor from the herbs, add to it a little Brandy, or camphorated Spirits of Wine. This is an excellent bath to strengthen the limbs; it removes pains proceeding from cold, and promotes perspiration.

Pierre-Joseph Buc'hoz,
*The Toilet of Flora* (1772)

As we have discovered, in the sixteenth and seventeenth centuries bathing had been viewed with suspicion or even trepidation. However, by the middle of the eighteenth century thinking was beginning to change. Medical opinion had shifted to advocating regular bathing as both therapeutic and hygienic, and the developing interest in personal hygiene had fuelled enthusiasm. From a therapeutic point of view, aromatic baths and visits to enjoy the rich mineral waters in places like Bath in England were deemed particularly beneficial. However, it was only the aristocracy who could afford to 'take the waters' in fashionable Bath, and systems weren't really in place for the ordinary public to have a regular bath at home. For a start, very few homes had taps or running water. Getting enough water to take a bath at home and then heating it sufficiently was not straightforward either.

Of course, there were baths and then there were *baths*. The wealthy, like French socialite Madame Tallien (1773–1835), could luxuriate in a bath of strawberries and scented milk. Even if the poorer classes had the opportunity to bathe, they would not be able to experience a soak in the most exotic herbs and spices. In his book *A Tour through several parts of England AD 1705*, Samuel Gale (1682–1754), the founder of the Society of Antiquaries in London, describes the benefits of the spa in Bath. According to Gale, upper-class ladies were able to bring their perfumed accoutrements with them while they took the waters: 'The ladies bring with them japanned bowls or basins, tied to their arms with ribbons, which swim upon the surface of the water, and are to keep their handkerchiefs, nosegays, perfumes, and spirits, in case the exhalations of the water should be too prevalent.'

## Soap and Water (Scented, of Course)

At London, and in all other Parts of the Country where they do not burn Wood, they do not make Lye. All their Linnen, coarse and fine, is wash'd with Soap. When you are in a Place where the

Linnen can be rinc'd in any large Water, the Stink of the black soap
is almost all clear'd awa'y.

François Maximilien Misson,
*M. Misson's Memoirs and Observations*
*in His Travels over England* (1719)

By the beginning of the eighteenth century the use of soap was
on the increase. However, it was still more likely to be used
for cleaning clothes and household fabrics such as tablecloths
than one's person, and as a commodity it was heavily taxed.
The cheapest soap was black soap, a mixture of lime and pot
ash. This was an almost liquid substance sold in small barrels or
firkins. Towards the end of the century, hard soap or white soap
made from lime and soda, bought in cakes or bars, became more
common. The French chemist Nicholas Lablanc (1742–1806) had
advanced the production of soap in 1789 by finding a way to
convert salt into soda, though his discovery was overshadowed by
the French Revolution.

Meanwhile, in Britain, by 1784 soap by law could only be sold
in cakes or bars, meaning that it had to be of a firmer consistency.
American statesman Benjamin Franklin (1705–1790) was given
the following soap recipe by his sister, who lived in England:
'eighteen bushels of ashes, one bushel of stone lime, three pounds
of tallow fifteen pounds of the purest Barbary wax of a lovely
green colour and a peck of salt'. While there is some attempt to
make this soap look more attractive, there is little effort to cover
up its strong smell. But scented soap could be made at home
using basic white soap, shaving it, reconstituting it and perfuming
it with things like rose, lavender, coriander, cloves, jasmine,
cinnamon, nutmeg, lemon peel, lemon juice, orange flower water
or musk.

Scented waters were among the bestselling products in the
major cities of Europe, most notably London and Paris. Scented
waters formed part of a lady's toilette and might be applied
directly to the body as well as to clothing. These waters were

also added to food and drink to enhance the flavour. As such these are found in contemporary recipes for cakes, creams, syrups and preserves. Scented waters were also taken internally for medicinal purposes. Pierre-Jacob Buc'hoz in his book *The Toilet of Flora* recommends a sweet-scented water consisting of a mix of rose water and orange water as 'an excellent perfume, and taken inwardly, is of service in some nervous cases and languors'. The French barber Jean Jacques Perret (1730–1784) refers specifically to the use of scented waters by men in his book *The Art of Learning to Shave Oneself* (1770), in which he recommended applying perfumed toilet water to the face after shaving 'to improve and temper the skin'.

Rosewater remained the most popular of scented waters, and although it could be purchased readymade many continued to make it at home – with an inevitable variation in strength and quality. Orange flower water was also in vogue and second only to rosewater in popularity. This was produced using neroli, an essential oil extracted from oranges. Although the best oranges were grown in France and Spain and imported into Britain, orange essential oil was also brought into Europe from the British West Indies at this time. As well as its use as a toilet water, orange flower water was a popular ingredient in cookery, skin lotions and cosmetic creams. Stored in dark blue glass bottles to hide the volatile liquid from the light, it was thought to aid digestion and calm the nerves as well as being regularly used to perfume sheets and linen. Again, according to Buc'hoz, 'the use of Orange Flower Water is very extensive. It is high in esteem for its aromatic perfume; and is used with success for hysteric complaints'.

Lavender water was another popular choice in the eighteenth century. Not only was it fashionable, but lavender water also had the advantage of being a somewhat cheaper option; by the turn of the century it was common to hear street sellers calling, 'Sweet lavender six bunches a penny.' In his 1788 book *The New Art of Cookery*, Richard Briggs, who described himself as 'many years cook at the globe tavern fleete street the white hart tavern

Holborn and the temple coffee house', includes the following recipe: 'Put two pounds of lavender pips in two quarts of water, put them in a cold still and make a slow fire under it; distil it off very slowly into a pot till you have distilled all your water: then clean your still well out your lavender water into it and distil it off slowly again; put it into bottles and cork it well.'

## Gloves and Handkerchiefs

> Take ambergris a drachm the same quantity of civet and orange
> flower butter a quarter of an ounce; and rub them into the gloves
> with fine cotton wool pressing the perfume into them.
>
> Robert Turner (1787)

The French guild of glove and perfume makers that had been established back in the middle of the previous century was formally disbanded as perfume became a product in its own right. Across Europe, however, this did not affect the popularity of gloves, nor did it have an impact on the need for gloves to be scented. Glovers, like a wide variety of other retailers, sold perfumed goods alongside their main product, including perfumed tablets, pastilles, hair powders, soap and fragranced cosmetics. Perfumed gloves were still considered de rigueur, particularly for ladies of good social standing. There was emphasis on the importance of keeping one's hands white and soft; some even wore gloves to bed for this purpose. Newspapers such as *The London Gazette* carried advertisements for premises that specialised in perfuming gloves, though perfumes houses such as L. T. Piver, founded in France in 1774, offered this service too. The waxy perfume could be applied to skins before they were made into gloves, or they could be scented when worn.

The handkerchief had become a very popular accessory by now, probably due in part to the increasing use of snuff; one took the snuff and sneezed into one's handkerchief. Also, women wafted their scented handkerchiefs in the air as a greeting much in the way that men doffed their hats. Handkerchiefs were valued not only as symbols of wealth and status (Louis XVI of France objected to anyone possessing a handkerchief larger than his) but also as love tokens and a means of flirtation; the scent that emanated from them served to reinforce these ideas. There were other options for wearing fragrance too. In the first half of the eighteenth century, fresh flowers carried in a nosegay or attached to the stomacher of a lady's dress (the triangular front panel) were popular. In the second half of the century scented ribbons arranged in a rosette and pinned to one's dress or tied around a nosegay were all the rage.

## Scented Homes and Fragranced Food

Keeping the bedroom fragrant was as important as ever to ward off insects such as bedbugs and nits, and in grand houses servants would treat bedheads to prevent infestations of bugs. The English cookery writer Hannah Glasse (1708–1770) went so far as to recommend that servants attach 'ash boughs and flowers' to the bedheads. Tansy was a popular choice for this purpose. Another option was to take the time to sew camphor into the mattress itself. Herbs grown in the garden such as lavender and lemon verbena were dried, put into small bags and kept among the linen and in clothes cupboards to keep garments fresh; from a hygiene point of view this was particularly important for linen underclothes.

The first known record of potpourri, meaning an aromatic mixture, is hardly a positive one. Lady Luxborough (1699–1756), in one of her epistles to fellow poet William Shenstone from 1749, writes of potpourri as 'a potful of all kinds of flowers which are severally perfumed and commonly when mixed and rotten smell very ill'. There is an element of personal preference when it comes to smells, of course, and perhaps Lady Luxborough preferred a simple rather than the compound mixture.

In the latter half of the eighteenth century pastille burners were lit to lend a space a pleasant aroma. Rather than being made of metal as they had been in previous times, eighteenth-century burners tended to be crafted from porcelain, often in the shape of miniature houses. The mixture placed in these burners consisted of powdered charcoal (often from willow wood) mixed with saltpetre which helped the mixture burn, along with a binder such as gum Arabic and lastly the all-important scent, an essential oil such as lavender, rose or cedar. The burner would be lit with a spill, a supply of which would be kept ready at hand.

Exotic scented fountains featured at grand dinner parties, and even artificial flowers brought in for the occasion might be scented to add to their appeal and give a sense of realism. Flummery, a sweet pudding rather like a blancmange or jelly, was a common sight on the dinner tables of the well-to-do, and rosewater or orange flower water was one important ingredient in this dessert. A decoration of edible fragrant flowers, such as nasturtiums, added to the appeal of fancy cakes and desserts. According to Hannah Glasse in her book *The Art of Cookery*, 'You may perfume the icing with what perfume you please.' Cookery writer Henry Howard in his book *England's Newest Way in All Sorts of Cookery* (1710) gives the following recipe under the heading 'a perfume to perfume any sort of confections': 'Take musk the like quantity of oil of nutmeg infuse them in rosewater and with it sprinkle your banqueting preparation and the scent will be as pleasing as the taste.'

## Scent Bottles, Vinaigrettes and Vanity Cases

Although eighteenth-century perfumes might be alcohol based, there were also those that were water based or wax based, which meant that the consistency of the final product still ranged from solid to liquid. However, liquid scent was becoming much more common, a factor which influenced the types of vessels used as containers. Other important influences on the shape and design of perfume vessels included whether the perfume was one a person would carry with them or whether it was for use inside the home. Perfume bottles could still be an indication that the owner had considerable financial means and, moreover, an appreciation of art and fashion. Decorative scent containers could be made of glass or rock crystal as well as porcelain, silver, gold, ivory or alabaster.

The chatelaine, a set of short chains usually attached to a woman's belt, in this period often held the keys to a home, indicating wealth. However, in the eighteenth and into the nineteenth century, a lady attending a ball might have a scent bottle attached to her chatelaine. The Chelsea porcelain factory made small containers for soft paste perfumes known as 'toys'. Crafted in a variety of shapes including human figures, animals and fruits, these were extremely popular as simple gifts or as tokens of love.

The vinaigrette was a box much smaller than its predecessor, the pouncet box, and was generally made of silver. It might be engraved, monogrammed or plain. Inside it held a sponge doused in perfumed oil with an alcohol or vinegar base. The scented sponge was fixed in place under a metal grille. The whole thing was small enough to fit into a pocket or a muff and could therefore be quickly taken out and the perfume applied when encountering a bad smell. Indeed, to do so was an expected part of contemporary etiquette. The ability of chemists to produce a more concentrated vinegar base had enabled the change from the heaver pouncet box to the lighter, more portable vinaigrette.

Large vanity cases, or nécessaires as they were known, had room for whatever a fine lady or gentleman might need if travelling, including a considerable number of perfume bottles alongside cosmetics (powders and paints) and other toilette implements (such as combs and brushes). The nécessaire became a popular wedding gift too. Much smaller vanity cases called etuis, intended to fit into a pocket, were another must-have item. These were also used as containers for other items such as sewing kits and writing tools. A perfume etui was likely to contain a small bottle or bottles of perfume, perhaps with a funnel for easy decanting. Etuis made of silver or semiprecious stone such as agate could be enamelled or covered in shark skin (known as shagreen).

Bouquet or posy holders, which had first become fashionable at the French court of Louis XIV, caught on as a fashion among the upper classes in early eighteenth-century Britain. Made from pearl, pinchbeck (a mixture of copper and zinc that resembles gold), tortoiseshell, silver or gold and sometimes encrusted with precious stones including diamonds, these holders contained a small posy that both disguised the owner's potential bad hygiene and protected them from exposure to unpleasant smells. They were considered a very suitable gift even for royalty. According to an issue of *The Times* from 1789, on the occasion of a visit from the Prince and Princess of Wales to a London workhouse, 'As [the coach] entered, a little girl came up and handed in a nosegay of flowers for the Princess. These were in a silver "handle", a tiny vase, which the paupers had paid for, and which was inscribed in Danish, "To Her Royal Highness the Princess of Wales from the 1,369 paupers and schoolchildren in Islington Workhouse."'

## Snuff, Tobacco and Smelling Bottles

> The snuffbox and smelling bottle are pretty trinkets in a lady's pocket and are frequently necessary to supply a pause in the conversation and on some other occasions. But whatever virtues they are possessed of they are all lost by a too constant and familiar use. And nothing can be more pernicious to the brain or render one more ridiculous in company than to have either of them perpetually in one's hand.
>
> Eliza Heywood, *The Female Spectator* (1745)

Snuff boxes and smelling bottles were certainly part of the eighteenth-century social scene and that only became more true as the century progressed. According to Miss Heywood, at least, it seems that these objects were as ubiquitous and potentially annoying as the mobile phone can be today.

Men smoked tobacco while women, and the more foppish of men, used snuff. In the eighteenth century, perfumers sold snuff or powdered tobacco. Snuff could be scented with the likes of rose or myrtle. In an anonymous poem from 1761 entitled 'Six reasons for taking snuff' we find reason for its use expressed more lyrically:

> When strong perfumes and noisome scents
> The suffering nose invade
> Snuff the best of Indian weeds
> Its salutary aid.

Women also carried smelling bottles containing either simple smelling salts (an ammoniac substance, spirit of hartshorn) or a perfume. The sight of a smelling bottle suggested not only femininity but a delicacy and frailty deemed fashionable for women at this time. It is also at this time that scent quickly develops a reputation as a means of reviving a fainting female. *Pharmacopeia Bateana, or Bates Dispensatory* (1706) describes Royal Essence – a mixture of musk, civet, balsam of Peru, clove oil, rhodium oil, tartar, salt and cinnamon – as both an 'odoriferous water' and a 'cure for fainting fits'.

In his travel book *A Tour through the Whole Island of Great Britain*, Daniel Defoe (1660–1731) refers to this increase in popularity in both snuff and smelling bottles when he lists the accessories required by a lady when visiting the spa in Bath sometime between 1724 and 1727: 'A handkerchief and a nosegay and of late years snuff box and smelling bottles are added.'

## Eau de Cologne

The first eau de cologne to bear the name was created by W. Johann Maria Farina (1685–1766). Johann's brother Giovanni Battista Farina had set up a fashion company in Cologne, and after Johann joined the business in 1714 the company, under his guidance, produced a citrus-based perfume that reflected the popular shift away from the heavy musk scents of the previous century. The scent was described by Johann Farina himself as 'like an Italian spring morning after the rain'. The list of ingredients was extensive: lemon, orange, tangerine, bergamot, lime, grapefruit, neroli, lavender, rosemary, thyme, petitgrain, jasmine and tobacco. Eau de cologne was marketed by the Farina brothers as a panacea for all ills, 'a miraculous antidote against poisons of all kinds and an outstanding prophylactic against plague'.

## Madame de Pompadour and Marie Antoinette

Members of the aristocracy placed much value on perfume; some of them still even preferred to supervise the preparations of their favourite scents. Perfume remained one of the largest expenses in a wealthy household, and among those who spent the most was Madame de Pompadour (1721–1764), mistress of Louis XV, King of France. Madame de Pompadour not only purchased perfume for herself, she also supported the perfume industry in general by founding the Sèvres porcelain factory, which became famous for its exquisite perfume bottles. Madame de Pompadour was also involved in launching Johann Maria Farina's citrus-based eau de cologne and marketed her own scented vinegar in 1740.

Marie Antoinette (1755–1793), the somewhat infamous wife of Louis XVI, had her own personal perfumer in the person of Jean Louis Fargeon (1748–1806). Both Marie Antoinette and Fargeon believed that scent should reflect something of the soul of the person who wore it. The queen had a particular love of floral scents and no doubt welcomed, or indeed even influenced, the move away from heavier musk scents. However, Fargeon did use musk in Marie Antoinette's favoured floral scents as a preservative, and it should be borne in mind that these floral substitutes would have been pretty powerful in their own right and perhaps not the delicate scent we might imagine today.

Marie Antoinette's love of perfume extended to scented gloves, bath sachets and the use of potpourri and other forms of room perfume in the palace. Just like the story that grew up around the capture of Catiline and his co-conspirators back in ancient Rome, after the French Revolution broke out the fleeing Marie Antoinette is alleged to have been discovered at the village of Varennes on the night of 20–21 June 1791 because her pursuers could smell her perfume. She is also understood to have taken three vials of perfume by the esteemed house of Houbigant (she loved their scents, especially eau de mousseline and eau de millefleurs) to the guillotine; whether to give her courage or to shield her from the odour of the Paris mob we cannot say.

## Napoleon and Josephine

In the latter years of the eighteenth century, perfume, far from being tainted by its association with pre-Revolution excess, survived and flourished. Though no doubt some businesses went to the wall, it had lost none of its appeal among those who had escaped the guillotine. Emperor Napoleon and his wife Josephine both adored perfume. Napoleon ate cologne on sugar, and under his rule the Palace of Versailles was scented with a mixture of aloeswood, sugar and vinegar burnt in vessels in the rooms. However, the otherwise adoring couple did not see eye to eye when it came to personal fragrance. Napoleon, who ordered fifty bottles of cologne per month, liked the scent of jasmine. Josephine, on the other hand, favoured the strong scent of musk, which her husband deeply disliked. She even had a following of musk-loving young men called Muscadins. However, the empress also favoured the scent of fresh flowers, particularly violets and mignonettes, both more in keeping with the general trend in perfume use at this time.

## The First Perfume Houses

The eighteenth century saw the establishment of the first perfume houses that made and sold their own branded goods. Their products were recognisable by their smell, of course, but often even before that by the shape of the bottle and the distinctive label attached to that bottle. At the top end of the scent market both the bottle and the label were designed to match the exclusive nature of their contents. These were works of art in their own right.

Floris was the first of these perfume houses to become established. Juan Floris, a Spaniard who had come to London to seek his fortune, opened his shop in Jermyn Street in London in 1730. Originally a barber and a supplier of combs, Floris and his English wife Elizabeth branched into scent with great success. Endowed with royal patronage, the company supplied luxury perfumes to well-to-do men and women. One of the company's early successes was the refreshing Limes perfume, which can still be purchased today.

Floris was followed into the perfume trade in 1775 by Jean Francois Houbigant, who established his shop at 19 rue du Faubourg Saint-Honoré in Paris. A glover, perfumer and supplier of bridal bouquets, Francois Houbigant was licensed as a member of the glovers and perfumers guild 'to make and sell all kinds of scents, powders, pomades, to whiten hands, cleanse the skin, soaps, toilet waters, gloves and mittens'. Houbigant's perfumes were distinctly floral and that association with flowers was firmly established from the very beginning and continues today; the company's logo has always been a basket of flowers. Houbigant's early fragrances included Evade, eau de mousseline, eau de millefleurs and eau de Chypre. Despite the upheaval of the French Revolution, Houbigant continued to thrive. Napoleon's war chest always contained a selection of Houbigant fragrances.

Colonial America entered the European perfume market with the founding of perfume selling enterprise Caswell Massey, originally an apothecary business. The company was established in 1752 in Newport, Rhode Island by a Scottish doctor named William Hunter. Caswell Massey became well known for its quality bath and hand soaps, apothecary remedies and shaving products. Hunter imported and blended his products by himself. Rather unimaginatively – though not unusually in the story of perfume, as the reader will discover – he simply numbered his scents as he created them and did not give them names. He produced numbers one to twenty, including cologne number six in 1789. This latter perfume contained cloves, orange peel, bergamot, orange blossoms and pine and was originally used as a wash for the hands and face. Number six was favoured by two early American presidents, George Washington and John Adams.

Maison Dorin (originally trading under the French name of Fards Rouges & Blancs ('make-up red and white') was established by Mademoiselle Montansier, an actress and businesswoman who brought flair and refinement to the cosmetics and perfumes that the business produced. In 1780 the company became the official supplier to the royal court at Versailles and, following the Revolution, began selling to more middle-class Parisiennes. Mademoiselle Montansier went into partnership with Jean-Marie Dorin, who renamed the company Maison Dorin after himself in 1819.

Creed, an exclusive British perfume house, was founded around 1760 by James Henry Creed. One of the first perfumes it produced, in 1781, was called Royal English Leather and was created in honour of George III, who took a particular shine to a pair of scented gloves he received from the company. A high-status brand, the company is still in the hands of the Creed family, who proudly use the tagline 'From father to son since 1760'. Not only did George III patronize the perfume house, but later Queen Victoria did too, along with a host of other royals and film stars.

L. T. Piver was established by Michel Adams in Paris in 1769. The company began selling perfumed gloves but by 1774 was manufacturing perfumes too. L'Essence Vestimentale, a lavender-based scent, was one of its first successes. A supplier to the court of Louis XVI, Adams' business adopted the name L. T. Piver when a young apprentice by that name eventually took over the company in 1813. The firm still exists today. Piver had a passion for Egypt, producing Eau de Pyramids to celebrate Napoleon's expedition to the Nile, and the company would follow up the theme of Ancient Egypt again in the nineteenth century when it launched Vallee des Rois in celebration of the discovery of Tutankhamen's tomb in 1926.

Andrew Pears (1766–1845), a barber by trade, opened his London shop in Soho in 1789. At first he specialised in selling make-up on the premises, in particular cosmetics that could cover up the damage done by the caustic soap that many were still using on their persons. Finally he branched into making his own soap, a product which was of a much lighter nature, based on glycerine with a fresh, flowery scent.

At the very end of the eighteenth century, Pierre Lubin, who had learned his craft from Marie Antoinette's personal perfumer Jean Louis Fargeon, established his perfume shop named boutique de roses in Paris in 1798. He specialised in perfumed ribbons, ball masks and scented rice powders, and first found favour with the dandies of Paris (known as the *incroyables*) and their fashionable companions the *merveilleuses*, the trendsetters of the day. More conventionally, Lubin found favour with Empress Josephine and with Napoleon's sister Pauline. In the nineteenth century the company added many of the crowned heads of Europe to their clientele.

## *Recipes*
### Lily of the Valley Scent

> Gather your Lilley-of-the-Valley Flowers, when they are dry, and pick them from the Stalks; then put a Quarter of a Pint of them into a Quart of Brandy, and so in proportion, to infuse six or eight Days; then distil it in a cold Still, marking the Bottles, as they are drawn off, which is first, second and third, &c. When you have distill'd them, take the first, and so on to the third or fourth, and mix them together, till you have as strong as you desire; and then bottle them, and cork them well, putting a lump of Loaf–Sugar into each Bottle. N.B. This serves in the room of Orange–Flower–Water, in 'Puddings, and to perfume Cakes; though it is drank as a Dram in Norway.
>
> Richard Bradley, *The Country Housewife or Ladies Director* (1728)

## A Perfumed Basket

Place a layer of perfumed cotton extremely thin and even on a piece of Taffeta stretched in a frame; strew on it some Violet Powder, and then some Cypress Powder; cover the whole with another piece of Taffeta: nothing more remains to complete the work, but to quilt it, and cut it of the size of the basket, trimming the edges with ribband.

Pierre-Joseph Buc'hoz,
*The Toilet of Flora* (1779)

## Syllabub Whipt

Take a pint of White-wine, and a pint of Black Cherry Juice, or Mulberry Juice; put into a large wooden Bole, sweeten it well with good white Sugar, put in also a great perfume Comfit, add to it a pint of Cream, make a rod of peel'd Willow, put to it a

Branch or two of Rosemary stript from the Leaves, wind about the rod a Limon-peel; after you have stirr'd the WIne and Cream well together whip it till it froths; take off the froth with a spoon, and put it into your Glasses; between every Layer of froth squeeze in some of the Spirit of Limon-peel; let if stand a Day after it is made before it is eaten.

William Salmon,
*The Family Dictionary* (1710)

## French Flummery

Take a Quart of Cream, and half an Ounce of Isinglass, beat it fine, and stir it into the Cream-Let it boil softly over a slow Fire a quarter of an Hour, keep it stirring all the time; then take it off the Fire, sweeten it to your Palate, and put in a Spoonful of Rose-water, and a Spoonful of Orange-flower Water, strain it, and pour it into a Glass or Bason, or just what you please, and when it is cold, turn it out. It makes a fine Side-dish. You may eat it with Cream, Wine, or what you please. Lay it round baked Pears; it both looks very pretty, and eats fine.

Hannah Glasse, *The Art of*
*Cookery Plain and Easy* (1747)

## Hair Pomade

Oil scented with Flowers for the Hair. Salad Oil, Oil of Sweet Almonds, and Oil of Nuts, are the only ones used for scenting the hair. Blanch your Almonds in Hot Water, and when dry, reduce them to powder; sift them through a fine sieve, strewing a thin layer of Almond-powder, and one of Flowers, over the bottom of the Box lined with Tin. When the box is full, leave them in this situation about twelve hours; then throw away the Flowers, and add fresh ones in the same manner as before, repeating the operation every day for eight successive days. When the Almond powder is thoroughly impregnated with the scent of the Flower made choice of, put it into a new clean Linen Cloth, and with an Iron Press extract the Oil, which will be strongly scented with the fragrant perfume of the Flower.

Pierre-Joseph Buch'oz, *The Toilet of Flora* (1779)

## Scented Pastilles

To form scented Pastils, roll up bits of this Paste in the shape of a cone that they may stand upright, and set them by to dry. These kinds of Pastils are lighted in the same manner as a candle. They consume entirely away; and, while burning, exhale a fragrant smoke

Pierre-Joseph Buch'oz,
*The Toilet of Flora* (1779)

## A Perfumed Soap

Take four ounces of Marsh-mallow Roots skinned and dried in the shade, powder them, and add an ounce of Starch, the same quantity of Wheaten Flour, six drachms of fresh pinenut Kernels, two ounces of blanched Almonds, an ounce and a half of Orange Kernels husked, two ounces of Oil of Tartar, the same quantity of Oil of Sweet Almonds, and thirty grains of Musk: thoroughly incorporate the whole, and add to every ounce, half an ounce of Florentine Orris-root in fine powder. Then steep half a pound of fresh Marsh-mallow Roots bruised in the distilled Water of Mallows, or Orange Flowers, for twelve hours, and forcibly squeezing out the liquor, make, with this mucilage, and the preceding Powders and Oils, a stiff Paste, which is to be dried in the shade, and formed into round balls. Nothing exceeds this Soap for smoothing the skin, or rendering the hands delicately white.

Pierre-Joseph Buch'oz,
*The Toilet of Flora* (1779)

## Snuff

Take some Snuff, and rub it in your hands with a little Civet, opening the body of the Civet still more by rubbing it in your hands with fresh Snuff; and when you have mixed it perfectly with the Snuff, put them into a canister. Snuff is flavoured with other perfumes in the same way.

Pierre-Joseph Buch'oz,
*The Toilet of Flora* (1779)

## To Candy Cowslips of Any Flowers or Greens in Bunches

Steep Gum-Arabick in Water, wet the Flowers with it, and shake them in a Cloth, that they may be dry; then dip them in fine sifted Sugar, and hang them on a String, ty'd cross a Chimney that has a Fire in it: They must hang two or three Days 'till the Flowers are quite dry.

Mary Eales,
*Receipts* (1718)

## Sweet-scented Washballs

Take of the whitest new Castile soap as much as you think proper; Scrape or grate it and then temper it with rosewater: thus set it for eight days in the sun; then add to it a few grains of musk and by stirring it about reduce it to a thick paste of which you may form excellent wash balls'.

G. Smith, *The laboratory or School of the Arts* (1799)

# 8

# THE NINETEENTH CENTURY
## Victorians, Violets and Synthetics

Won't you buy my sweet blooming lavender?
Sixteen branches one penny
Ladies Fair makes no delay
I have your lavender fresh today
Buy it once, you'll buy it twice
It makes your clothes smell sweet and nice
It will scent your pocket handkerchiefs
Sixteen branches for one penny.

Victorian street cry

By the nineteenth century the cities of Europe were not only overcrowded but also choked with smog, the air dirtied with the often toxic emissions generated by the new industrial society. Until the 1890s and the advent of germ theory, the idea that 'bad air' (miasma) caused disease would prevail, so air quality was a serious concern. Novelist Charlotte Bronte (1816–1855), describing a visit to fellow writer Elizabeth Gaskell's house in 1851, gives us a sense of the way in which the scent of flowers could make living in the towns and cities more bearable. She describes the house as 'a large cheerful airy house quite out of the Manchester smoke. A garden surrounds it and as in this hot weather the windows were kept open a whispering of leaves and perfume of flowers always pervade the rooms.'

As if the fumes from industrialisation were not enough, horror of horrors, the stench in Paris was compounded by the smell from a leaking graveyard. In the late eighteenth century, the walls of a burial ground known as the Cemetery of the Innocents had crumbled, allowing decaying human remains to spill into the cellars of those who lived nearby. The foul smell in Paris became known as 'the Big Stink', and pleasant fragrances were deemed essential in the effort to protect the city's inhabitants. There was a growing market for perfumes in America, too, where many people lived in cities where the air was contaminated by the smell of gasworks, slaughterhouses and general waste. Perfume was still a vital tool in the struggle against these noxious smells. French perfumes were still highly valued, and Paris remained the centre of the universe as far as scent was concerned, while the town of Grasse was its industrial hub.

## Scent and Gender

While men as well as women continued to wear scent, particular perfumes were now deemed more suited to one or the other. That is to say, in this century gender appropriate scent began to replace the previous trend of mostly blanket usage of whatever an individual chose as a preference regardless of their sex. The trend was floral for women while more 'masculine' scents (aromatics like sandalwood for example) were worn by men. It was still the general rule that when respectable people wore perfume they applied it to their clothing and their accessories rather than directly onto their skin. Both men and women might opt for a perfumed handkerchief, for example. A gentleman could wash with Brown Windsor soap (a mixture of bergamot, caraway, cinnamon and clove) and might inhale scented snuff. Perfumed buttonholes were a must for the well-dressed gentleman too. A lady would, as matter of course, use a wide variety of scented products as part of her daily toilette. Particularly when venturing out, she might wear a corsage, carry a small perfume bottle on her person, perhaps in a small handbag or, as it was known a reticule. A lady might even have scent sachets sewn into the fabric of her dress. In fact, she might perfume her clothing even down to the buttons on her dress.

It is safe to say that for women in particular, perfume was a consideration when it came to clothing. Fragrant or aromatic smelling salts remained a must to revive ladies when feeling faint or ill. The tight corsets which were the fashion of the day no doubt caused much of the fainting phenomena, which was frequently commented upon, though no doubt feigning a faint could be manipulated to the lady's advantage should she want to escape present company or alternatively draw the attentions of an admirer. As had often been the case in the past, fashionable clothing could not easily be washed. The heavy dresses worn by upper- and middle-class ladies had to be sponged down, sprinkled with eau de cologne, toilet water, attar of roses or perhaps violet powder in an attempt to remove stains and conceal any bad odours.

## The Variety of Scent

Aside from a fragrance to wear on clothing or to daub on accessories, scent still came in many different forms, from potpourri to pastilles, perfumed snuff and tobacco, and was used for many different purposes. There were scented sachets to keep clothing smelling fresh while in storage, as well as fragranced syrups to add to desserts, aromatic toothpastes, breath fresheners (known as cachous), smelling salts and soaps, the latter scented with rose, almond or orange flower. The range of perfumed cosmetics, aimed largely at women, was extensive too and included powders, lotions, creams for the face and scented products for the hair. To quote from *The Scientific American* (1862), 'Starch becomes Violet Powder, soap becomes Old Brown Windsor, glycerine becomes crème de mauve ...water is impregnated with elder flowers and fat is inoculated with orange blossoms.'

There were some strange inventions too. One such product was called Papier d'Armenie. This was manufactured in Paris at the behest of French politician Auguste Henri Ponsot (1877– 1963) and prompted by his visit to Armenia, where he witnessed the burning of styrax resin mixed with aromatics being used to fragrance and disinfect the home. Small sheets of paper were soaked in this mixture and it was sold in little booklets. In short, many otherwise basic commodities were perfumed. Once a mundane product was impregnated with a scent, it became much more desirable.

Perfumed goods could be purchased at varying prices not only in store but also, thanks to the development of postal services, by mail order. The vast number of retail outlets selling scent and the option to order by post, together with the fact that America began to play a much more important role in the market for perfume at this point in our story, all combined to broaden the consumer base.

## Books, Magazines and Trade Catalogues

Perfume continued to be much written about. Etiquette guides such as the *Ladies Book of Etiquette and Manual of Politeness* by Florence Hartley (1860) and *Gems of Deportment* by Martha Louise Rayne (1881) are but two examples of this genre. Titles like these advised on how to behave, what to wear and how (and when) to wear it. Regular catalogues produced by individual perfume houses as well as the new department stores showed off the variety of fragrances available. These catalogues were posted out to customers often free of charge. Books about gardening contained information about making your own scents, which was still a popular pastime. Housekeeping manuals and regular weekly or monthly magazines included instructions as to how to make your own fragrances at home too. The increasing number of new magazines (especially those aimed at a female audience) advertised particular brands of perfume available to buy in the shops and gave hints and tips on the latest fashions in fragrance.

Much of the content of these magazines was aimed at the middle classes, who wanted to copy the style – in perfume as in everything else – of the fashionable society ladies.

There was no shortage of technical manuals for the professional perfumer either. *The Art of Perfumery*, written by the London perfumer G. W Septimus Piesse (1820–1882), co-owner of the prestigious perfume business Piesse and Lubin, was first published in 1855 and had already run to a third edition by 1862. This was a particularly important tome as it established the idea of perfume 'notes' (top, middle and base), a terminology founded scientifically on the evaporation time and intended use of each scent. The term is still in regular use today.

## The Popularity of Lavender and Violet

> The fondness for violets increases with time and many women of fashion will tolerate no other fragrance.
>
> *American Soap Journal and*
> *Manufacturing Chemist* (1895)

Exclusive perfumes purchased from both the established and new perfume houses were far from cheap. However, there were respectable alternatives. Simple eau de cologne (in its original meaning, rather than its modern sense of a particular strength of scent) was a citrus-based toilet water that was popular and relatively inexpensive. Lavender too was a ubiquitous, cheap scent that was well-liked by all classes. The cries of lavender sellers like the one quoted at the beginning of this chapter echoed around the streets of eighteenth-century towns.

Eliza Doolittle is the central character in the play *Pygmalion*, written by George Bernard Shaw (1856–1950) and the basis for the film *My Fair Lady*. Doolittle is first introduced to the theatre and film audience as a poor flower girl selling violets. Girls like Eliza would have been a common sight in the nineteenth century as well as the early twentieth century. Violets were very popular despite the fact that their flower was associated with melancholy in the era's so-called language of flowers. Particular flowers had been endowed with certain meanings since at least Shakespeare's time, but it was the Victorians who truly codified this. Despite this association, violets proffered a particularly appealing fragrance that was used in perfumes and toilet waters as well as soaps, tooth powders and cosmetic sachets for scenting clothes. According to an 1898 edition of *The Spatula*, a trade magazine for pharmacists, one could even purchase 'a soft thick violet coloured flannel which exhales the most delicious perfume ... The flannel is cut into strips and sewed into the linings of sleeves waists and skirts and into the crowns of hats and bonnets.'

Worn by both men and women, violet's scent was much in demand in Europe and continued to be popular into the beginning of the twentieth century. However, if one had some status in society then the scent should not be derived from just any old violets. According to an edition of the *New York Herald* from the eve of the twentieth century, 'While violet is the perfume of the season ... it is quite common for dainty women to have their own individual perfume formulated as they fancy it should be – for there are violets and violets.' Certainly advertisements appeared in nineteenth-century media for all sorts of different types of violet scent, implying that these perfumes were derived from violets of particular geographical origins. There were Russian violet perfume, Rhine violet perfume and San Remo violet to name but a few. One Margaret Gainer stole a bottle of violet perfume from a hairdresser's shop; she clearly felt the scent was worth some sacrifice, because she refused to return it and therefore served a thirty-day jail sentence. Even with what seems such an innocent scent, however, it was a case of *caveat emptor*. The *British Medical Journal* in 1880 reported on a case involving the death of an infant:

> The jury returned a verdict that she died from blood poisoning from the application to the body of an irritant containing sulphate of lime ... which was sold by the chemist as violet powder.

Mignonette, a flower with a scent similar to violet, was popular for scenting the home. According to the horticulturalist Henry Philips (1779–1840), writing in 1830, even those who were overwhelmed by the smell of mignonette indoors would be 'delighted with the scent it throws from the balconies into the streets, giving breath of garden air to a close-pent man'.

Aside from violet, lavender and mignonette, rosemary, bean flower, strawberry and heliotrope were also very much in favour, as were jasmine, rose and honeysuckle. The purple garden flower heliotrope, with its light and powdery fragrance, was particularly popular during the latter half of the nineteenth century. The following piece, taken from an 1840 edition of *The Saturday*, a weekly journal, gives the reader a sense of the nature and range of scents available at the time, and the uses to which they were put:

> Herbs, drugs, and flowers, are made to yield their aromatic odours for our use. Among the former we may mention marjoram, sage, thyme, lavender, &c., while of drugs, frankincense, mace, cloves, benzoin, storax, and many others, are held in great esteem. Orange-flowers, jonquils, jessamine, roses, violets, and other fragrant flowers, are also largely employed, and thus, by a judicious use of some of these various essences, we may impart to our dwellings or our dress, the delightful odours of our favourite flowers, at any period of the year.

## Delicate Perfumes

> A perfume should be so delicate, so daintily used, and so lingeringly fragrant that no one could define it as any thing but the ghost of a sweet scent, a faint, clinging memory of sweetness.
>
> Martha Louise Rayne, *Gems of Deportment* (1881)

For wealthy women, delicate floral scents were very much in fashion. It was important to conform on this matter, as the choice of perfume could still give a clue to one's social status. London perfumer and marketing expert Eugene Rimmel (1820–1887) in his *Book of Perfumes*, first published in 1865, made the connection between choice of perfume and status very clear, advising women to use 'simple extracts of flowers which can never hurt you in preference to compounds which generally contain musk and other ingredients likely to affect the head. Above all avoid strong coarse perfumes. A woman's good taste and good breeding may as easily be ascertained from the perfume she uses.' According to one article on perfumes from the American magazine *Godey's Ladies Book* (1850), 'as a first principle all decided or strong odors are in bad taste. What is a perfume but the counterfeit breath of sweet flowers and nature rarely overdoes her work.'

However, though perfume for the upper-class woman should be delicate in accordance with contemporary fashion, it was certainly laid on quite thick if *Gems of Deportment* is any true indication:

A handkerchief, a glove, a veil, or any article of a lady's dress should be so permeated with the fine fragrance of the toilet as to be inseparable from herself; but not a suspicion of cologne. Lubin's extracts, or Price's sweet violet should attach to her. This is only attained by a constant use of the same fine perfumes in liquid or sachet form. Her trunks are perfumed, her gloveboxes, her mouchoir case, her bonnet box, even her shoes. Her hairbrush is sprinkled with rose-water or a more delicate perfume, and in this way she gets the balm of a thousand flowers so condensed and directed that it becomes her own individual perfume.

While the scent in itself may have been subtle, it would not have been difficult to create an overpowering effect if a lady were to perfume every item of her dress, accessories and accoutrements as this passage suggests.

## *Strong Scents*

> An ingenuous reviewer once described some verses of mine
> as 'unwholesome' because he said they had 'the faint smell of
> patchouli about them'.
>
> Arthur Symons (1865–1945)

In her *Manuel des Dames*, French author Madame Elizabeth Celnart (1796–1865) takes her disapproval of strong perfumes one step further than Eugene Rimmel had done, remarking that 'strong odours such as musk, amber, orange blossom and tuberose and others of this kind are strictly forbidden'. Strong perfumes were said to reflect an immoral lifestyle and were regarded with suspicion. Patchouli, for its part, was admired at the beginning of the nineteenth century, but it experienced an interesting rise and fall. The enthusiasm for patchouli was fuelled by the fashion for fine imported Indian shawls, which arrived in Europe duly scented with the fragrance. Fashions changed, as they inevitably do, and in the middle years of the nineteenth century, when Arthur Symons was writing, patchouli had developed an association with less reputable women. All was not lost, however, and within a few decades patchouli had reinvented itself as an acceptable fragrance for men.

Despite the trend towards light florals for women, some still enjoyed stronger odours such as ambergris, musk and civet, so these did not disappear altogether. Indeed, the company Viner saw a market for stronger scents as well as lighter ones, appealing to both preferences in their advertisement for fragrances for the gentleman's waistcoat and for the ladies reticule or handbag: 'Rose, violet, musk, tonquin, mareschal … verbena geranium, forget me not and patchouli.'

At any rate, because musk and other animal-derived scents were used as fixatives in perfumes where other, more floral smells predominated, there was still a market for these ingredients. Indeed, the respected perfumery house Piesse and Lubin advertised themselves as importers of both musk and ambergris. However, besides those who disliked the strong smell of these perfumes there were others who objected on grounds of animal cruelty. Obtaining musk was a distressing process as far the animal was concerned. As a result, on ethical and moral grounds, as well as changing fashions and personal preference, the use of genuine musk was fast becoming history.

## Perfume and Medicine

> All should read this. During the prevalence of Typhoid Fever, Bubonic Plague, Cholera, and Small Pox. Do not fail to have packets of 'PETAL DUST,' freely distributed in the house, under the bed and in chests of drawers, wardrobes, in the folds of bed linen, and every place where clothes are kept ... DECREASE OF THE PLAGUE IN INDIA. Thousands of Packets of 'PETAL DUST' are distributed daily in the plague stricken districts.
>
> Nineteenth-century newspaper advertisement

Petal dust was manufactured by the Rosemarine Manufacturing Company and sold as a floral air purifier and an everlasting perfume. However, in the advertisement quoted above the key selling point is its strength as a medicine. There is nothing particularly strange about this. Perfume and medicine, as we know, were long-time bedfellows. Indeed, this connection continues to the present day in the form of aromatherapy. However, the link would never be as close as it had been in the past. In fact, among the groups who would call perfume to account in the nineteenth century were doctors and psychiatrists who thought that scent might make neurotic individuals even more unstable. According to French chemist and physician Dr Rostan (1790–1866), 'hysteria, hypochondria and melancholia are its most usual effects'. Others, among them the poet T. S. Eliot (1888–1965), expressed a similar opinion: 'Again the insistent sweet perfume and the impressions it preserves irritate the imagination or the nerves.' We know now that, aside from mere preference, some people are very sensitive to particular smells, or even allergic.

Opinions on the value of scent as a medicine and prophylactic varied. Many still saw the medicinal and psychological benefits of a pleasant smell. Despite the loosening of the connection between scent and medicines, in comparison with past centuries, the influential Eugene Rimmel for example was still advertising his popular toilet vinegar as a cologne that 'sprinkled on a pad hung up in the air destroys bad smells and noxious effluvia in sick rooms closets etc'. The following advertisement appeared in various newspapers including the *Morning Post* in 1807: '[J Delacroix] respectfully informs the nobility gentry and public that he has prepared a vegetable vinaigre de toilette of the salubrious herbs and roses.' A toilet vinegar was in fact strong aromatic vinegar, a cologne tended for use principally as a skin cleanser, aftershave and mouthwash, but as this product was 'salubrious' and potent against 'noxious effluvia' it was also intended for use in maintaining good health.

One particularly important development in the relationship between perfume and medicines is encapsulated in a decree from 1810 by Napoleon wherein he stipulates that pharmaceutical and chemical manufacturers must display their goods separately from perfumes and soaps at trade exhibitions and must also list their ingredients. Perfumers, meanwhile, were not required to disclose the ingredients they used; divulging the make-up of a product could destroy some of its mystery and allure. As a result, perfume businesses like the new House of Guerlain could experiment with fragrances without having to disclose their ingredients to the competition.

Interestingly, the decree also specified that anything defined as a perfume should not be consumed internally. At the time there was some concern among the medical profession that ladies whose status forbade them from frequenting public houses instead drank perfume for its alcohol content, creating a serious risk to their health. One Dr Meredith, in his book *Recollections of a Country Doctor* (1885), challenges a patient on noticing there is little left in her scent bottle: 'If that eau de cologne has been spilt on the table it would have left a mark on the polish ... Why keep this sort of humbug? Why not tell me you have drunk it?'

## Dandies and Decadents

Perhaps surprisingly, the famous dandy Beau Brummell (1778–1840), the man who almost singlehandedly dictated men's fashion in the early part of the nineteenth century, seems not to have worn scent so much on a day-to-day basis. Instead he was scrupulous about hygiene. However, in order to achieve the level of cleanliness he sought, Brummell would have made use of scented soaps, perhaps a lighter shaving cologne, and tooth powder, which would also have been scented.

Though shunned to an extent by the fashionable Beau Brummell, perfume did become closely associated with contemporary art and in particular with the decadent lifestyles of a group of mostly young male artists and writers known as the Decadents. The group included the playwright Oscar Wilde (1854–1900), poets Charles Baudelaire (1821–1867) and Arthur Symons (1821–1867) and the artist Aubrey Beardsley (1872–1898). Association with these men was unlikely to give perfume a good name; their hedonistic and depraved behaviours went against Victorian morality, even if that morality was often little more than a veneer. The poet and civil servant Theodore Wratislaw (1871–1933) observed, 'Oscar joined me spraying himself with a scent which filled the room. I inquired its name: "It is white lilac," he said, "a most insidious and delightful perfume."' The artist Aubrey Beardsley went so far as to spray the flowers in his garden with opoponax and frangipani.

In a similar vein, in France we come across the poet, essayist, art critic and dandy Robert de Montesquiou (1855–1921), a member of the Symbolist art movement, which sought to imbue lines, colour and form in contemporary art and literature with a deeper symbolic meaning. Famously acquainted with and painted by the artist James Whistler, the aristocratic de Montesquiou held receptions in his Paris home. Each room was an artistic experience, painted in a different colour and scented with a different perfume. The Symbolist movement was instrumental in encouraging olfactory elements in theatre performances too. While this had been done before, the Symbolists went further. Even theatre programmes were scented, having been carefully stored in boxes between perfumed sheets awaiting distribution to the audience as they arrived.

## Mechanisation and Invention

Since 1878 the substitution of mechanical work has increased again producers use steam, alembics, infusing devices, extracts, shaker's grinding and pulverising machines, hydraulic presses, pomade mixers, saponification boilers a whole range of devices specific to toilet soaps designed for shaving perfume and mixing colours grinding moulding casting packing.

Alfred Pickard, 'Report of the Universal Exhibitions' (1891)

In a work entitled *The British Perfumer, Snuff-manufacturer, and Colourmans Guide; being a collection of choice receipts and observations proved in an extensive practice of thirty years* (1822), published posthumously on behalf of Charles Lillie, the author dismisses homemade scents as 'scraps of old women's receipts ... gleaming from table talk'. In contrast, this was the age of industrialisation, mechanisation and subsequently mass production. The Industrial Revolution brought about many changes in the way people lived and worked. It revolutionized the perfume industry too. By the middle of the century, steam power had become crucially important in speeding up the manufacture of scent, helping to increase production and bring down prices. The result was that more and more people could afford scented goods that had in the past for the most part been luxury items.

Consider soap production as an example. This became both cheaper and much faster. Businessman Alphonse Honore Piver (1812–1882) patented the 'automatic dryer', which turned plain soap into scented soap in the space of a few days rather than taking over a month. A gentler, more fragrant soap was mass produced for personal use in contrast to the harsh caustic product that had largely been used for cleaning one's clothes. Chemical solvents were used in the treatment of fragile flowers, and perfume accessories once regarded as essentials were superseded; for example, the invention of the atomiser meant perfumed fans fell out of fashion.

## The Science of Synthetics

The nineteenth century saw the invention of alchemical substitutes for natural scents. These are known collectively as aldehydes. Their importance was acknowledged at the time by George William Askinson in his work *Perfumes and their Preparation* (1892):

> The great progress which the art of perfumery has made during recent times is due to several causes ... the advance in our knowledge of the physical and chemical properties of the several substances used in perfumery ... Synthetic chemistry has also added to the list of materials required by the perfumer, and is surely going to add many more to it hereafter...

A whole array of chemical substitutes was developed in the nineteenth century which, no doubt, reflects the number of scientists working in this field and the importance of scent as a functional and desirable product, both economically and socially. One of the first of these synthetics was produced in 1833. Named eugenol, it simulated the smell of cloves. Substitutes for cinnamon (cinnamaldehyde), anise (anethole), bitter almonds (benzaldehyde) and heliotrope (heliotropin) were also among the early chemical substitutes to be discovered. By the end of the century the chemists had even managed to produce a synthetic replica of the sought-after fragrances of both jasmine and rose.

Although violet was a particularly popular scent in Victorian times, to make a perfume from the real thing required a lot of flowers and could be expensive. According to the pharmaceutical journal *The Spatula*, 'violet perfume may be extracted from the flowers themselves but one hundred pounds of violets produce only one ounce of the finest extract'. In her journals, Queen Victoria describes visiting a perfume factory in Grasse where she and her daughter Beatrice were conducted through 'several large corridors which were literally carpeted with Parma violets and yellow jonquils to a room where women were at work throwing masses of violets into boiling lard'. The smell was 'too delicious'.

To get around the sheer number of violet flowers needed to make even a small amount of perfume by the latter years of the nineteenth century, this scent was likely to be created using synthetic materials too. In 1893, two German chemists, Ferdinand Tiemann (1848–1899) and Paul Krüger (1859–1916), developed a synthetic substitute that they named ionone after the Ancient Greek word for violet. Incidentally, ionone is also the name of the nymph who was said to have stolen the secret of perfume from the goddess Aphrodite and given it to Helen of Troy.

Other synthetics mimicked less obvious fragrances. The synthetic coumarin, for example, replicated the smell of fresh hay. The perfume house Houbigant was the first to use this chemical in its famous scent Fougère Royale, a nineteenth-century perfume that is still on sale today. Until the end of the twentieth century, coumarin was also added to cigarettes. This is no longer the case, and the synthetic compound is now banned from use as a food additive in the United States. However, it can still be found in shampoos and soaps in the twenty-first century. Jicky, a perfume first manufactured in the Victorian era, would become a prime mover in the following century and combined synthetic ingredients with orris, bergamot and lavender oils. The scent was a favourite of the actress Sarah Bernhardt (1844–1923).

Among the many scientists on the trail of the elusive synthetic scent was the German chemist Albert Baur (1836–1933), who, in 1888, stumbled upon an artificial alternative to musk quite by accident while he was trying to make, of all things, an explosive. Bauer's synthetic musk was in fact a derivative of TNT, and this toxic creation has now fallen out of use.

While the notion that art could improve on nature had previously been an unthinkable concept, in the nineteenth century it had become an acceptable idea. The theory that man could better nature was expounded by, among others, the caricaturist Max Beerbohm (1872–1956) and the French novelist Joris-Karl Huysmans (1848–1907), whose book *A Rebours* (*Against Nature*), published in 1884, extolled perfumes made from synthetics as 'a fabulous counterfeit of the countryside'. Due to this change of heart, there was little objection to chemicals that replaced natural ingredients. Synthetic substitutes for the real smell of flowers, animal secretions and herbs were hailed as a wonderful success. There were good practical reasons for this too. Perfume from plants and animals were both costly and difficult to produce in large quantities. Using synthetics was more cost effective and allowed supply to more easily meet demand as well making it easier to create a product with longer-lasting fragrance, which had always been a challenge. It seems that, when science allowed, all thought of the superiority of nature was set aside in favour of substitutes valued for their cost and stability.

## Naming a Perfume

Although some scents were simply named after their main ingredient (violet or white rose, for example) or perhaps simply given a number, others bore names that ranged from the regal to the provocative, the floral to the sporty, the fun to the romantic and the exotic to the commemorative. Some would have been considered rather risqué for their time, like Stolen Kisses (1861) or Kiss Me Quick (1873), both by Piesse and Lubin. In their chosen names, these perfumes openly acknowledged the sexual allure of scent. Others celebrated an event. Piesse and Lubin launched their Leap Year Bouquet by advertising it with the witty rhyme, 'In the leap year they [women] have the right to choose. Ye men no charter to refuse.'

The cachet of a French name, with its connotations of luxury and romance, had not gone out of fashion and it was not only French companies that exploited these associations, as with Fantasia de Fleur by Creed and Parfum d'Arabie by Poole. In 1855, perfume maker Breidenbach of New Bond Street, London targeted a male audience with perfumes sporting labels such as Royal Hunt and Newmarket Jockey Club. Even his floral scents were advertised for men: one advertisement reads, 'Breidenbach recommends all sporting gentlemen to try his wood violet perfume on sale at various prices.' Other manufacturers also appealed to a male audience, invoking the lifestyle of an upper-class gentleman in their names: Guards Club Bouquet and the Belgravia (both L. T. Piver) and the Oxford and Cambridge Bouquets (Metcalfe, Bingley and Co.). Clearly scent was an accoutrement expected of any gentleman.

## Commemorative Scents

In the second half of the nineteenth century in particular, there was a fashion for celebrating all sorts of events with the creation of a new perfume: a royal wedding, an important exhibition, or a discovery of historic significance. The death of the explorer David Livingstone (1813–1873) prompted the manufacture of the Livingstone Bouquet (in 1873). The Alexandra Palace Bouquet was launched in 1875 to celebrate the reopening of the Alexandra Palace following a fire. We see the beginnings of the concept of celebrity scent in the Sarah Bernhardt Bouquet, named after the popular actress of the era and launched in November 1880. Bernhardt had been a sell-out in her New York show and tickets had gone on sale for her London performances. Maker Eugene Rimmel simply cashed in, proving that he was a man with excellent business acumen.

Royal marriages were always a popular reason for celebration and worthy of a new scent to commemorate the event. The Romanoff Bouquet went on sale in 1873 in honour of the marriage of the grand duchess Marie Alexandrovna of the Russian imperial family to Queen Victoria's son Prince Alfred, Duke of Edinburgh. Even the latest novel might be marked by the launch of a new perfume. One example of this is Little Dorrit's Nosegay, which was produced in celebration of Charles Dickens's novel and advertised in *Bell's Life in London, and Sporting Chronicle* in the Christmas of 1855.

## Personalised Perfume

> The scene was dazzlingly brilliant to me as I entered. The grand
> staircase and ante-chamber were decked with garlands, and
> festoons of white and gold muslin and ribbons. The blaze of
> lights, the odour of flowers, the perfumes, the diamonds and the
> magnificent dresses of the cream of the British aristocracy smote
> upon my senses;
>
> Lady Isabel Burton (1831–1896)

What better way to announce your arrival at a prestigious social gathering, such as the one at which young Lady Burton found herself, than to wear your own exclusive perfume? Queen Victoria herself patronized the perfume house of Creed, so in 1845 the company presented her with a personalised scent which they named Fleur de Bulgaria, a mixture of Bulgarie rose, from which took its name, mixed with musk, ambergris and bergamot. This must have been quite a heavy, sensual perfume for a lady with such a prim reputation to wear, perhaps hinting that our stereotypical view of the queen is likely inaccurate.

Empress Eugene (1826–1920), a Spanish aristocrat and the glamorous wife of Napoleon III (1808–1873), was also a devotee of Creed. In 1860 she had a particular cologne made for her called Jasmin Imperatrice Eugenie, a light perfume consisting of lemons, oranges, bergamot, lavender and rosemary – in short, a floral scent with a hint of the exotic. This scent is still on sale today in the original bottle design, with French bees stamped on in real gold dust. Eugene's influence on the world of fragrance did not stop there. She persuaded Creed to move its headquarters from London to Paris so that it would be close at hand for her.

The scent Floris 127 was another personalised perfume, first made in 1890 for Grand Duke Orloff of Russia (1869–1927). The duke was an advisor to Tsar Nicholas II and, after the Russian Revolution, an influential émigré with more than a passing interest in fragrance. Floris noted in its ledger that the scent was for Orloff alone. They were true to their word: the formula was not sold to anyone else until after his death.

## Fictional Scents

> The studio was filled with the rich odour of roses and when the light summer wind stirred amidst the trees of the garden there came through the open door the heavy scent of the lilac or the more delicate perfume of the pink flowering thorn.
>
> Oscar Wilde, *The Picture of Dorian Gray* (1890)

The Decadents as a group were strongly influenced by Huysmans' *A Rebours* with its descriptions of olfactory excess and praise of artificiality fitting well with their flamboyant dress and lifestyle. More specifically, Huysmans' seminal text is thought to have been the inspiration for Oscar Wilde's famous and disturbing novel *The Picture of Dorian Gray*. In Wilde's book perfume plays a central role, expressing the depravity and eroticism so fundamental to the storyline. The eponymous character Gray researches perfume and is obsessed with its power: 'There are flowers in every room and furniture made of scented wood upon which is placed perfume for handkerchiefs.'

French novels featured perfume too: there is scented soap in *Cherie* by Edmond de Goncourt (1822–1896), a novel about

French feminine adolescence, and a pomade of jasmine in Emile Zola's (1840–1902) *Le Ventre de Paris*. Zola, like Wilde, was interested in the effects of perfume. But Wilde expressed a preference for almond blossom scent, believing that strong perfumes could be dangerous. In poetry, perfume was popular not only as a principal subject but also to convey ideas central or peripheral to the understanding of the verse. Charles Baudelaire in his work *The Immorality of Scent* played on the musical connotations established scientifically by Piesse: 'As others minds sail, on the crest of music mine floats, on the waves of your perfume.' Baudelaire's erotic collection of poems entitled *Les Fleurs du Mal*, which took perfume as its subject, was considered shockingly provocative at the time but would eventually result in the launch of an actual scent bearing his name in 2009, a leathery fragrance by Byredo. The sexual connotations of scent are exploited to the full here much as they are in the toilette scene in Oscar Wilde's play *Salome* (1891). Zola's novel *Nana*, the story of a cheap prostitute's path to high-class call-girl, is another example of conveying meaning through scent: 'In the muggy air intermittently lingered a more acute odour; it was coming from a few sprigs of dried patchouli broken into tiny pieces at the bottom of a glass.' The mention of patchouli, with its aforementioned connotations at the time, implies Nana's station in life. Virginia Woolf (1882–1941) deplored cheap perfume, while Herman Melville (1819–1891) in his celebrated novel *Moby-Dick* mused on the value of ambergris: 'Who would think, then, that such fine ladies and gentlemen should regale themselves with an essence found in the inglorious bowels of a sick whale?'

## Painting Scent: John Collier, Alma Tadema and Floral Asphyxiation

The idea that one could be fatally overcome by the fragrance of flowers had been mooted in Roman times and was recalled in a nineteenth-century work by the Dutch artist Lawrence Alma-Tadema (1836–1912). His painting *The Roses of Heliogabalus*, completed in 1888, is a visual representation of a scene from the life of the Roman Emperor Heliogabalus (*c.*AD 203–222) preserved in a collection of late Roman biographies known as the *Historia Augusta.* Alma-Tadema painted the story of a legendary banquet held by the emperor where the attendees were showered with flowers. Many of the guests, overcome by the scent, supposedly died. The beautiful painting takes on a somewhat sinister hue when the viewer understands that the people in the picture are dead or dying.

Floral asphyxiation became something of a trope in nineteenth-century art and literature. It featured in Zola's novel *The Sin of Father Mouret* and in John Collier's (1850–1934) painting *The Death of Albine* (1895). The two undoubtedly influenced each other, portraying the same story in different media. Albine, an innocent girl left heartbroken after an unfulfilled love affair, dies, according to Zola, 'completely buried under hyacinths and tuberoses'. Works of art and literary descriptions representing asphyxiation in this manner beg many questions. Are these images disturbing or beautiful? How do we react to them? Do they remind us of sleeping beauty, passive and peaceful, or do they conjure up more sinister thoughts?

Whether there were any actual examples of such a thing happening in real life is unclear. However, in the nineteenth century flowers were not considered healthy in sickrooms. This was in marked contrast to times past when roses, violets and other pleasantly fragranced flowers had been not only a cover-up but a cure for bad odour and disease. Suffice to say, the now traditional gift of flowers to someone in hospital or at home unwell would not have been appreciated at this time.

Despite these rules during sickness, once deceased it was common for a person to be surrounded by flowers in the Victorian era. We see flowers in abundance on coffins or in photographs of the dead in repose. Photographing the dead may be difficult for a modern audience to understand, but we can appreciate the practicality of the flowers given that in the Victorian era the corpse might lie in the house for several days after death. Flowers, perfumes and scented candles were not only decorative but served their more functional and long-established role of covering the unpleasant smell of decomposing flesh.

The erotic nature of scent, a theme we have already acknowledged in contemporary literature, also appears in nineteenth-century art. *Fumée D'ambre Gris*, a canvas painted in Tangiers in 1879 by the American artist John Singer Sergeant (1856–1925) and first exhibited in 1880, still stuns with its representation of the intoxicating, sensual nature of scent. We can see the wisps of ambergris rise from the fretted brazier with its burning coals. The painting contrasts the purity of the woman in white and the animal quality of ambergris itself.

This is to say nothing of the stage. On arrival, members of the audience might be presented with a scented theatre programme. Just like the performance they had come to observe, the audience was also there to be seen. The women in particular dressed up for the occasion, and that included donning their best perfume. At the première of *The Importance of Being Earnest* in 1895, Oscar Wilde commented on the fact that 'nearly all the pretty women wore sprays of lilies against their large puffed sleeves while rows and rows of young elegants had buttonholes of the delicate bloom of the lily of the valley'. Such sights and smells would certainly have pleased Wilde.

## Scented Letters, Valentines, Fountains and Finger Rings

> A plain paper, heavy, and of a clear, cream white is the Best for social and domestic correspondence … Very dainty young Ladies affect a pink tinted paper and violet perfumed ink, upon which basis they begin a gushing correspondence with six or eight school friends, wherein the adjectives suffer much harm.
> Martha Louise Rayne, *Gems of Deportment* (1881)

Not only theatre programmes but other forms of cards and papers might be impregnated with perfume to add to their romantic appeal. Sometimes romantically attached couples sent perfumed valentine sachets rather than cards. Letters might also be daubed with scent to rid the correspondence of any germs. French writer Alexander Dumas (1802–1870) in his unfinished novel *The Red Sphinx*, a sequel to *The Three Musketeers*, touched upon a rather more sinister reason for applying scent to a letter: to reveal a hidden message:

> Alone in her room, Anne of Austria listened to the receding footsteps of Gaston d'Orléans and of her mother-in-law … From a drawer she took out a small canvas bag containing iris powder, a perfume she preferred for her clothes above all others, and which her mother-in-law had brought her from Florence. This powder she sprinkled on the blank second page of the letter from Gonzalès de Cordova.

Sealing wax was perfumed with essential oils such as that of lavender, mace, cloves, rhodium, benjamin or ambergris. The presence of a scent in cheaper seal waxes was even more important because it helped to disguise the poorer quality of the resin used.

Following on from the Great Exhibition, held in London in 1851, perfume fountains became de rigueur at public exhibitions and events as well as balls and large society parties. At the opening of the Crystal Palace in 1854, Eugene Rimmel put out the following newspaper advertisement:

> Rimmel perfumer to Her Majesty 39 Gerrard Street, Soho, London will commence playing his perfume fountains for the accommodation of the visitors as follows; the Toilet Vinegar north east end, the Sydenham Bouquet south east corner of the great transept the Eau de Cologne south east end. These perfumes may be had on the spot at 1s and 2s a bottle.

Others, including Piesse and Lubin, also exhibited perfume fountains. Advertisements indicate that though men still used fragrance these installations were for the most part aimed at women. According to an 1858 edition of *The Morning Post*, 'ladies visiting London's Crystal Palace can have their handkerchiefs perfumed gratuitously in Rimmel's perfume fountain'. In Emile Zola's work *The Ladies' Paradise* shoppers are delighted by 'a silver fountain ... from which a continuous trickle of violet water was flowing, tinkling musically in the metal basin. An exquisite scent was spreading everywhere and the ladies soaked their handkerchiefs in it as they passed.' The fountain finger ring advertised by Piesse and Lubin was a more portable version of the same idea and sold as a great novelty: 'Useful, ornamental and a source of fun ... each ring will hold about half an ounce of scent and can be filled with the greatest of ease all at a cost of one shilling and sixpence.'

## Shopping for Scent

Scents purchased at the many perfume houses were exclusive and therefore, inevitably, expensive. The fashionable perfume boutiques in the centre of nineteenth-century Paris exuded opulence, their fashionable interiors in keeping with the goods on sale: elegant furniture, large windows with display cabinets and expensive wood counters, mirrors, pots and scales. The decor was sometimes augmented by water features and plants. The Houbigant boutique in Paris was faithfully restored to its 1885 elegance in 1955 and included ornate counters, showcases and chairs in lemon tree wood, expensive parquet flooring and an elaborately decorated ceiling.

High prices often served to make products look more desirable and luxurious, but in the nineteenth century they varied greatly. Scented toilet soaps, pomades, oils, lotions and eaux de cologne could be purchased more cheaply away from the more exclusive houses. In France, from the 1850s onwards, the new department stores began to open their doors. The most famous among these are Le Bon Marché, which opened in 1852, followed by Grands Magasins du Louvre in 1855 and La Samaritaine in

1870. However, these shops did not immediately open perfume departments and though perfumed goods were advertised in their shop catalogues at this stage they did not receive particular prominence as they did not account for a large portion of department store sales. Instead, many exclusive fragrances remained merchandise sold in glamorous perfume boutiques. However, alongside department stores, which began to give perfume more prominence in the 1880s, by the 1890s perfume bazaars began to flourish, offering a large range of cheaper products. These bazaars had stands open to the pavement and served customers from nine o'clock in the morning until at least ten o'clock at night, giving ample time to purchase their wares.

## Packaging the Product: Selling the Dream

> In the space between the stands and the window arrange neat
> boxes of perfumes, or anything suitable for presents.
>
> *The Chemist and Druggist* (1896)

Newspapers, magazines, trade cards and handbills continued to be a means of promoting your scented wares. The nineteenth century also saw paper fans, scented cards, sachets and sample bottles aimed at men as well as women and given away to customers to entice them back to buy the full product. In 1871, Freeman Ballard Shedd (1844–1913), an American philanthropist who had made his money in pharmaceuticals, began producing cards soaked in a scent called German Cologne to give it extra appeal. Shedd's German Cologne was aimed at the male market, and his cards were given out as samples for advertising purposes. By the end of the nineteenth century, aside from scented promotional material, a whole range of items in daily use might be perfumed including calendars and even train timetables.

Competition in what was an ever-expanding market meant that presentation, while it had been important as far back as ancient times, took on even more significance. As more and more scented goods were shop bought, the packaging could not only echo the quality of the goods themselves but also help to quickly identify the product and distinguish it from the many others on sale.

Boxes, caskets, bottles and the like were intended not only to entice the buyer to purchase but also to evoke and sell an idea or an emotion, whatever that might be: love and romance, power and wealth, a memory or a mystery, perhaps. Take the Rothesay bouquet for example. This scent was advertised as 'the most fragrant and lasting perfume for the handkerchief' and sold in one-shilling or two-shilling bottles according to the Bute Post Office directory of 1893. Rothesay, the main town on the Isle of Bute in Scotland, was a popular holiday destination in the nineteenth century so it was fitting that the place had a perfume named after it to sell to visitors as a souvenir that would recall the memory of their visit.

No doubt engraved and coloured labels on perfume bottles drew the attention of the buyer, identified the product and also added to its appeal and ultimately helped to justify the high price. Better printing technology allowed for greater use of colour, enabling the production of decorative labels that suitably mirrored the luxury, quality and sophistication of the product. This early advertising established motifs associated with various perfumes and perfume houses that have been sustained to the present day, such as Houbigant's basket of flowers. The decoration and style of perfume bottles would continue to develop as an art form, with the best artists commissioned to design labels. Scents produced by L. T. Piver had labels engraved by the famous Sèvres porcelain factory for example.

Piesse and Lubin advertised toilet bottles for the mantelpiece – that is, pieces worthy of being put on show. Many were pricy items set with gems, becoming desirable objects in their own right long after their contents had been used up. In 1862, covering Piesse and Lubin's display at the London Exhibition of that year, *Scientific American* acknowledged the importance to the market of fine perfume containers: 'The manufacture of gold, silver and aluminium smelling bottles to contain smelling salts is of no mean importance as a branch of the jewellery trade.'

## America

'Oh no,' said a chemist, 'it does not follow nowadays because a toilet perfume is made in France or any other foreign country that it is superior in quality to one of American preparation. Such was formerly the case but the art of making fine perfumes has been carried to such perfection of late years. In this country that not more than one eighth as much of the French preparations is sold in the United States today as was sold ten years ago.'

*The New York Sun* (1885)

Wealthy Americans copied trends in Europe, picking up on the continental obsession with perfume use as part of social etiquette. American men and women carried scented handkerchiefs. Women held or wore nosegays, and men sported buttonholes (also known as boutonnières). Devotees of French and English scents, the Americans would also create more of their own in this century, of which Florida water was the standout product. At last, America had its own perfume. This citrus-based cologne was made from sweet oranges spiced with lavender, clove cassia and lemongrass. Invented in New York by the perfumer Robert I. Murray in 1808, Florida water was very popular in the United States with both men and women but did not really catch on elsewhere. The scent was enjoyed not only for its fragrance but was also believed to be beneficial against depression and temper exhaustion. According to *The Women's Book* of 1894, 'The perfume it leaves about her person will not be sufficiently powerful to cause discomfort to anyone.' Its name referred to the fountain of youth that according to tradition was situated in the state of Florida. No doubt the connection did the product no harm at all.

Theodore Ricksecker (1846–1919) is famous as one of the first major American-born perfumers. According to *The Merck Report* and *Pharmaceutical Journal*, 'Mr. Ricksecker is thoroughly original in his ideas and methods. He is also a clever artist and designer. This is seen not only in his ability to create new and effective blending of odours, but in the various bottles, boxes, labels, marks and advertising show cards, all of which designs emanate from his fertile brain.' He combined his skill as a perfumer with an eye for beautiful containers made of hand-painted porcelain that added to the appeal of his products. Who would not have wanted visitors to see these beautiful items on their dressing table?

## Famous Nineteenth-century Perfume Houses
### Guerlain
Guerlain opened for business in 1828 in the rue de Rivoli in Paris. Its founder, Pierre-François Pascal Guerlain (1798–1864), was a French chemist who had learned his trade in England. In 1834 at the Exposition des Produits de l'industrie Française, Guerlain showed off a number of scent products including Eau de Vie de Lavender, a rouge for cuts and bruises, Vinagrillon de Seville, intended as an air freshener; Poudre Sympathetique to scent paper and letters, and a more traditional pomade of bear's fat as well as perfume intended for soaking handkerchiefs named Bouquet de Roi. His clientele included Napoleon III and Queen Victoria as well as the Russian royal family, for whom he personalised his perfumes.

### House of Coudray
The company was founded in Paris in 1810 by doctor and chemist Edmond Coudray. Travelling all over to collect exotic plants and having won a number of awards at prestigious exhibitions, Coudray became a supplier of perfumes to the British court. His scents include Reine Victoria, created for the queen herself, as well as a fragrance named Gants Poudrés (Perfumed Gloves) and another called Rêve de Reine (The Queen's Dream). In 1828 Coudray also published a book entitled *Secrets de Beauté* in which he stated, 'The art of being beautiful ... is also the art of wearing perfume.'

## Crown Perfumery

Crown Perfumery was established in 1872 by American-born William Sparks Thomson (1823-1907) already a supplier of crinolines and corsets to European aristocracy. Though American, Thomson's business premises were to be found in London. As he was already known to the queen, she granted him permission to feature an illustration of her crown on his perfume bottles. The connection with royalty was an obvious selling point, and Thomson certainly understood the importance of presentation. His lavender salts became a bestseller, with buyers attracted not only by the finest lavender essence but also by the clearly identifiable dark green bottle. His crab apple blossom perfume, an entirely new fragrance, was also a great success.

## Grossmith

Founded in London in 1835 by one John Grossmith, the company was awarded a royal warrant by the British, Greek and Spanish royal families. Its most famous perfume, Phul-Nana (which in the Hindi language means 'lovely flower'), was promoted as 'a bouquet of India's choicest flowers'. The perfumes produced by the firm played into the European conception of the East. Grossmith's scents were for the very wealthy and came in various forms, including scented soaps and breath fresheners. An original bottle of Phul-Nana recently featured in the television series *Downton Abbey* as a gift to Violet Crawley, Dowager Countess of Grantham. While certainly accurate in terms of date, whether a lady as conservative as the dowager countess would have worn such a modern and sensual perfume is another question entirely.

## Rimmel

Eugene Rimmel (1820–1887) was the son of a scent manufacturer. His *Book of Perfumes*, first published in 1865, is an important contemporary source of information for this period. He claims that he was the first perfumer in England to employ female workers, appreciating them for their dexterity. In 1862, Rimmel was perfumer to both the Queen of Spain and the King of Portugal. As well as bottles of perfume he sold perfumed books, valentine cards, theatre programmes and even perfumed cushions, Christmas cards and Christmas crackers. He invented and patented the perfume vaporizer, which despite being a bit of an advertising gimmick was nonetheless used in theatre productions, for example in the early ballet *The Fairy Acorn Tree*, as part of the storyline and to create atmosphere, much in the tradition of Shakespeare's time.

### Piesse and Lubin

G. W. Septimus Piesse (1820–1882) and Pierre Francois Lubin (about whom very little is known) opened their shop on Bond Street in 1855. Among the scented products the firm sold, according to nineteenth-century advertisements, were 'toilet powders, odorous vinegars ... pomatums, scented oils, perfumed soap ... perfumes for the handkerchief, [and] scented waters'. Their list of concentrated flower essences and so-called 'primitive' mixed perfumes for scenting the handkerchiefs ran to around fifty different varieties. With exciting names ranging from the regal (Her Majesty's Perfume and Empress Eugenie's Nosegay) to the romantic (Cottage Flower and St Valentines Nosegay), Piesse and Lubin seem to have delighted in choosing names for their perfumes. Their Jolly Dog was immortalised in song, and they also manufactured the somewhat risqué Box His Ears. The company sold curios such as scented shells imported from the Maldives at 2 shillings per dozen as well as scented ribbons known as Ruban de Bruges, sachets of powders for use in babies' blankets, gift sets, and rose oil to conceal the smell of stale tobacco.

Bouquet Opoponax, first marketed in 1859, was a scent based on a sweet resin similar to myrrh and was one of the most popular products manufactured by the company. When the wreck of the *Mary Celestia*, an American Civil War blockade runner that sank in 1864, was discovered intact by divers off the coast of Bermuda, among its contents were two labelled and intact bottles of Bouquet Opoponax.

## Truefit and Hill

Established by William Francis Truefit, this London barbershop and perfume house catering to the well-groomed gentleman opened its doors in 1805 and still trades today. One of the company's first perfumes, developed in 1815, was intended to appeal to the stylish undergraduates at Oxford and Cambridge, and was aptly named Freshman. The company created the Palmerston Bouquet for the Prime Minister of the time and was patronized by royalty as well as other perhaps less reputable figures such as Oscar Wilde.

## Atkinsons

James Atkinson moved from the north of England to establish a factory in London where he could manufacture perfumed goods based on his own recipes, setting up shop in Bond Street in London in 1800. By 1832, Atkinsons (James had been joined by his brother Edward) had become an official court perfumer. The business became known initially for a quality traditional hair pomade, made from bear's grease, hence the company trademark of a bear. Atkinsons' first perfume was called British Bouquet, a tribute to the style of Beau Brummell. More traditionally, in 1837, James produced Bouquet de la Reine to celebrate the coronation of Queen Victoria. The company followed this with Nuptial Bouquet on Victoria's marriage to Prince Albert. A second wedding perfume called White Rose was manufactured for the royal wedding of trendsetter Princess Alexandra, who received a bottle of this scent every week for the rest of her life.

## Penhaligon's

Penhaligon's was the brainchild of hairdresser William Henry Penhaligon (1837–1902), who fell in love with the smells emanating from the Turkish baths close to his hairdressing establishment in the capital's Jermyn Street and decided to experiment and develop his own fragrances. He named his first – and very successful – scent Hammam Bouquet, the name alluding to its inspiration. The rest, as they say, is history.

## *Recipes*
### A Pomatum

Take 2 ounces yellow wax and 12 ounces beef marrow. Melt all together and, when sufficiently Cool, perfume it with the essential oil of almonds.

> John Marquart, *600 Miscellaneous*
> *Valuable Receipts, Worth their*
> *Weight in Gold* (1860)

### Eau de Cologne

To make Eau de Cologne: Rectified Spirits of wine, four pints; oil of bergamot, one ounce; oil of lemon, half an ounce; oil of rosemary, half a drachm, oil of neroli, three quarters of a drachm; oil of English lavender, one drachm, oil of oranges, one drachm. Mix well and filter. If these proportions are too large smaller ones may be used.

> Florence Hartley, *The Ladies' Book of*
> *Etiquette and Manual of Politeness* (1860)

### Morocco Snuff

Forty parts of French or St Omer tobacco with twenty parts of fermented Virginia stalks in powder; the whole to be ground and sifted to this powder add two pounds and a half of rose leaves in fine powder; and the whole must be moistened with salt and water and thoroughly incorporated. After that it must be worked up with cream and salts of tartar and packed in lead to preserve its delicate aroma.'

> Colin Mackenzie (ed.), *The British Perfumer,*
> *Snuff manufacturer and Colourman's*
> *Guide by the late Charlies Lillie* (1822)

## Flummery

Steep in cold water, for a day and a night, three large handfuls of very fine white oatmeal. Pour it off clear, add as much more water, and let it stand the same time. Strain it through a fine hair sieve, and boil it till it is as thick as hasty pudding, stirring it well all the time. When first strained, put to it one large spoonful of white sugar, and two of orange flower water. Pour it into shallow dishes, and serve it up with wine, cider, and milk; or it will be very good with cream and sugar.

> Mary Eaton, *The Cook and Housekeeper's Complete and Universal Dictionary* (1822)

## A Lavender Sachet

For a lavender Sachet: Ground lavender flowers 1lb, gum benzoin in powder half a pound, attar of lavender a quarter ounze

> G. W. Septimus Piesse, *The Art of Perfumery* (1857)

## Scented Soap

Cut the soap into thin shavings and heat it with enough water until liquefied. Let it cool to 135 degrees fahr., and add lavender flowers ground 1 lb: gum benzoin in powder ¼ lb; otto of lavender ¼ oz.

> Henry Hartshorne, *The Household Cyclopedia of General Information* (1881)

## Lavender Perfume for Smelling Salts

Six drams of oil of lavender aug., one dram, and half of essence of ambergris, two drams of essence of bergamot and a half of essence of musk. Mix and shake well before dropping on the salts.

> *The Girls' Own Paper* (February 1898)

## Hungary water for the Bath

Pure alcohol 2 quarts; essence of rosemary (Hungarian if possible) 28 grammes; lemon peel 14 grammes; essence of balm; mint 14 grammes; essence of peppermint; 4 grammes; extract of rose 28 centilitres; Mix and let stand for two weeks. The filter and it is ready for use.

> Harriet Hubbard Ayer, *A Complete and Authentic Treatise on the Laws of Health and Beauty* (1899)

## White Smelling Salt

Mix in a large porcelain jar—

Carbonate of ammonia 2 lb. Caustic ammonia 1 lb.

Cover the jar and leave it at rest. After some days the mixture will have changed into a firm mass of monocarbonate of ammonia which is rubbed to a coarse powder, perfumed, and filled into bottles. The above quantities require:

Oil of bergamot 15 grains. Oil of lavender 15 grains. Oil of nutmeg 8 grains. Oil of clove 8 grains. Oil of rose 8 grains. Oil of cinnamon 75 grains. The oils are poured into a mortar and rubbed up with about one-tenth of the salt; of this perfumed salt enough is added to the several portions of the mass, and triturated until the odor is equally distributed. For cheaper smelling salts oils of geranium and cassia may be substituted for the oils of rose and cinnamon.

> George William Askinson, *Perfumes and Their Preparation* (1892)

## Aromatic Vinegar

Concentrated acetic acid, 8 oz. Otto of English lavender, 2 drachms. rosemary, 1 drachm. cloves, 1 camphor, 1 oz.

First dissolve the bruised camphor in the acetic acid, then add the perfumes; after remaining together for a few days, with occasional agitation, it is to be strained, and is then ready for use.

Several forms for the preparation of this substance have been published, almost all of which, however, appear to complicate and mystify a process that is all simplicity.

G. W. Septimus Piesse, *The Art of Perfumery* (1857)

## Cachou Aromatise

Take of extract of liquorice and water each 3 ½ oz; dissolve by the heat of a water bath and add Bengal catechu in powder 462grs; gum Arabic in powder 231 grs. Evaporate to the consistence of an extract and then incorporate the following substances previously reduced to a fine powder mastic cascarilla charcoal and orris root 30 grs. Reduce the mass to a proper consistence remove it from the fire and then add English oil of peppermint 30 drops, tincture of ambergris and tincture of musk each 5 drops; pour on an oiled slab and spread it by means of a roller to the thickness of a sixpenny piece. After it has cooled apply some folds of blotting paper to absorb any adhering oil, moisten the surface with water and cover it with sheets of sliver leaf. It must now be allowed to dry and cut into very thin strips and these again divided into small pieces about the size of a fenugreek seed.

Henry Hartshorne, *The Household Cyclopedia of General Information* (1881)

9

# THE TWENTIETH CENTURY
## Cinema, Haute Couture and
## Celebrity Scents

The continued use of a good perfume is a mark of individuality.
By selecting a distinctive odour and using it constantly you create
a magnetism. For those who know you best that is fascinating.
Such was the custom if the court ladies of France before the
revolution and so it is today with the fastidious ladies of that
most sociable land.

*The Telegraph* (1906)

## Introduction
In the twentieth century, France set the fashion in fragrance
very much as it did in clothing. The town of Grasse was still
the centre of agriculture for this purpose, supplying the perfume
industry by producing huge amounts of fresh flowers from which
manufacturers extracted the precious essential oils. However, by
the end of the first decade of the twentieth century, perfumers
were experimenting with compounds made possible by the ever-
expanding range of synthetics available. In some cases, these were
used to replicate the smell of a real plant or animal substance. In
other instances, the smell was a new one all of its own. Mixed
together, different fragrances both real and synthetic could
produce a distinctive odour.

Readymade perfume was a thriving and lucrative commercial market which had begun to attract companies better known for more mundane products such as toothpaste and deodorant rather than high-end perfumes. Colgate, for example, ventured into perfumes as early as 1866 and within fifty years had become a big player in the industry with a total of 625 perfume lines listed, with names such as Carnival Violets, Lilac Imperial and Christmas Bouquet.

At the very beginning of the twentieth century, the fashion for light florals for women prevailed. For gentlemen, Guerlain's Jicky, launched in the latter years of the nineteenth century, was a popular choice. The fragrance possessed a musky leather scent that appealed to the male market. For the well-dressed gentleman, scented buttonholes were all the rage at this time. The orchid was the choice of King Alfonso of Spain (1886–1941), as well as the British Prime Minister Sir Neville Chamberlain (1869–1940). Macassar oil was popular in the Edwardian era and worn by men to style their hair. This was a mixture of oil (coconut or palm) and the scent of ylang-ylang. Guerlain's Mouchoir de Monsieur, which translates as gentleman's handkerchief, was an instant hit when it was launched in 1904. Originally created for the wedding of a family friend, Mouchoir de Monsieur was discreet but particularly long lasting when daubed on a handkerchief. However, the fashion for applying scent in this way was beginning to fall out of fashion.

Perfumes, especially those for domestic use such as room fragrances or linen fresheners, might still be made up at home from ingredients readily available in the shops. The *Dudley Recipe Book* (1910), compiled by society beauty Georgiana, Countess of Dudley (1846–1929), describes the following method of fumigating a room: 'Heat in the fire a long-handled scent fumigator, when it is red hot put into it some powdered cedar wood which can be bought at any store. This is preferable and far more agreeable than the heavy perfumes which are often used for this purpose.' The recipe clearly illustrates the ready availability of the ingredients to make your own air freshener, though there is no indication of cost. The long-handled scent fumigator would have been made of metal with a perforated lid to allow the aromatic smell to escape and fill the room. The passage also acknowledges the importance of personal preference.

Companies selling readymade soaps, household cleaners, room fresheners and the like needed to pay greater attention to the fragrance they added in order to make their product competitive and saleable, even at the cheaper end of the market. In the words of research chemist W. A. Poucher (1891–1988), whose textbook *Perfumes, Cosmetics and Soaps* (1923) is now into at least its tenth edition:

> Household products of a traditionally obnoxious nature are no longer in vogue, however, and the trend is towards the elegant presentation of even the most mundane commodities. An appealing perfume is often virtually essential for the success of the product. Woe betide any manufacturer who pays but scant attention to perfume when the public expects an attractive aroma!

By the 1920s, scent vending machines were a common sight. London Transport and the Automatic Amusement Company worked together to provide these in the city's railway stations, no doubt to their mutual financial benefit. In theatres and cinemas, alongside cigarette and sweet machines, scent machines dispensed luxury perfumes such as Evening in Paris by Bourjois, Shalimar by Guerlain and Quelques Fleurs by Houbigant. The scent came out of the machine in small vials called nips, made from a strong plastic called plastene. No need to worry if you had forgotten your perfume or were invited out on a surprise date.

## The Healing Properties of Scent

At the beginning of the century, scent retained little more than the vestiges of its association with medicine and health when compared with times past. However, in subtle ways it lingered.

There was still an understanding that smell could lift the spirits and support mental health, while some scented plants and resins were known to have a beneficial effect on a person's physical wellbeing too. Scented toilet vinegar was standard issue in first-aid kits at the beginning of the twentieth century. Roses were employed for their anti-inflammatory properties. Myrrh, recognised as a painkiller since biblical times, was also regarded as an effective antibacterial agent.

However, there were some practices around at this time involving scent that were definitely not good for one's health. Alarmingly, in 1912, *The New York Times* reported that women in Paris were injecting themselves not with 'morphia, cocaine or caffeine, they now employ as stimulant hypodermic injections of otto or rose and violet and cherry blossom perfumes. An actress was the first to try the new practice. She declared that forty-eight hours after the injection of the perfume known as "new mown hay" her skin was saturated with the aroma.' Thankfully, this idea did not catch on.

The question of the health benefits of smell, or at least scented flowers, came under greater scrutiny when the French chemist and scholar Rene Maurice Gattefosse (1881–1950) suffered an unfortunate accident, burning his hand in a laboratory explosion. Gattefosse immediately plunged his hand into the nearest liquid available, which just happened to be lavender oil. The chemist was taken aback at the healing effect that the oil had on what was a serious burn. The accident could have left major scarring but didn't, and he put this down to the lavender oil. He coined the word *aromathérapie* and published his classic work under that name in 1937, detailing within his definitive research into essential oils. Understandably, however, the discovery of antibiotics eclipsed his study and it was not until the 1950s that Austrian-born biochemist Marguerite Maury (1895–1968) pursued his research, providing personalised aromatics for her clients to suit their temperament and any particular health issues. According to Maury, 'perfumed essences when correctly selected represent medicinal agents'. By the end of the century many appreciated the potential health benefits of aromatics but alongside that appreciation there was a growing concern about use of fragrances, especially with reference to skin contact and allergies.

## The Changing Role of Women

From the early years of the twentieth century, women's lives had begun moving in a very different direction. There was a demand for change, first from the Suffragettes led by Emmeline Pankhurst (1858–1928), and later from the feminist movement in the 1960s. New technology and world events – particularly the two world wars – not only had a profound effect on the status of women but also brought about changes in the perfume they wore.

In 1900, the company Houbigant found the luscious silhouette of the Gibson girl an ideal vehicle for marketing their Le Parfum Idéal. The Gibson girl was a caricature drawn by the American artist Charles Dana Gibson (1867–1944) that represented a generic independent American woman with a narrow waist and prominent bust, a precursor of the Barbie doll. With the image of the Gibson girl on the label, Le Parfum Idéal, created for Houbigant by its joint owner Paul Parquet (1856–1916), was displayed at the Paris Exposition of 1900. It smelled like a bouquet of many different flowers including carnation, ylang-ylang, jasmine, Bulgarian rose and orange blossom, though in actual fact it was based on synthetic chemicals. This scent also evoked the continuing interest in the East as a source of fine perfume and significantly, in respect of the female gender, defined the wearer as not only independent but provocative – a sign of things to come.

However, alongside contemporary scents like Le Parfum Idéal with its more daring reputation, nostalgic florals like Yardley's English Lavender were still doing well. The traditional scent of violets was even linked with the Women's Social and Political Union, led by Emmeline Pankhurst. According to the National

Women's Party in the United States, as per a newsletter from 6 December 1913, 'Purple is the colour of loyalty, constancy to purpose, and unswerving steadfastness to a cause.' The Suffragettes were certainly audacious and innovative, but they did not sever their ties with all femininity.

For those of an even more adventurous nature, however, there arrived on the market a range of scents for women that were not only more daring but were also more masculine in composition. The first of these masculine scents for women was Tabac Blond by Caron, created in 1919, just a year after women secured the vote (at least for those over thirty) and the First World War had come to an end. Aware that women had experienced a newfound independence, including dispensing with their corsets, wearing trousers and doing jobs previously done by men, Caron offered women a change in fragrance that distanced itself from those Victorian and Edwardian feminine florals and even topped the more risqué scents available. Tabac Blond reeked of tobacco, and those bolder, more liberated women in society who smoked wore it with enthusiasm. However, though the scent went well with the fashion for bobbed hair, flapper dresses and the Jazz Age, it was not considered a scent for 'nice girls'. Tabac Blond was followed by other breakthrough scents, including Shocking (1937), created by fashion designer Elsa Schiaparelli (1890–1973). The perfume did just what it said on the label, being overtly sensuous in every way. The bottle which helped sell the brand reflected its content, modelled on the sultry figure of the outspoken film actress Mae West (1893–1980). The perfume's ingredients included civet, musk *and* ambergris, previously dominant in scents aimed at men.

The feminist movement helped to create a market for perfume with liberated sexual connotations. A fashion for patchouli re-emerged in the hippie era, the age of 'free love'. Both Charlie by Revlon (1973) and the American scent Baby Soft (1974) launched by Dana were great successes. There should perhaps be a word of caution here, however. Many people looking at the advertisements for Baby Soft with a twenty-first-century eye would find them more than a little distasteful. The scent, a powdery mixture of rose, jasmine, geranium and musk, was initially promoted with the tagline, 'Because innocent is sexier than you think.' This message, combined with images of preteen or adolescent girls, leaves a bit of a bad taste now. The company did, however, modify its marketing campaign and the product continued to sell well for many years.

Alongside the women's movement and the changing ideas and tastes that resulted, the structure of the perfume market itself was changing too. From the middle of the twentieth century, some of the big names in the perfume industry would be swallowed up by other businesses. By the 1960s Max Factor had taken over Corday, Caron was a public company and Yardley had become part of BAT industries. There were more affordable, less exclusive perfumes on sale too. However, the luxury market continued to flourish. Mass production in the seventies and eighties drew the criticism that poorer-quality scents were flooding the market. However, the more exclusive and better-quality scents were still there, albeit at eyewatering prices. Cheap and cheerful, it seems, was the order of the day. Poucher:

> Changes in the men's market have also partly been influenced by changes in the role of women within our society, in turn influenced in the latter half of the twentieth century by the fact that perfume became more and more of an everyday item available to everyone. It became a status symbol to own a luxury perfume with a fashionable name of the moment and to ask for it as a birthday or Christmas gift if too expensive for the recipient to buy.

Young girls were the target of Avon's Pretty Peach and Sweet Honesty. Many today remember the packaging with a certain fondness and would buy this scent today, such was its influence on young girls of an impressionable age.

A flourishing market emerged in perfume for men as well. New fragrances for men included Kouros by Yves Saint Laurent (1981) and Brut by Brut (1964). A *kouros* was a type of ancient Greek statue that represented the embodiment of flawless male youth. The name Brut has similar masculine connotations, of course. A further new trend developed soon after, in the nineties, with the arrival of Calvin Klein's CK One, a unisex scent intended as perfume for women and an aftershave for men. Developed in 1994, CK One was indicative of the growing sense of equality between men and women. Its simple bottle and packaging helped sell its dual image as well as addressing contemporary concerns about protecting the environment.

## Selling Scent

To add to the already existing commercial outlets, more and more department stores opened their doors to customers at the beginning of the twentieth century. Among them was Selfridges in London's Oxford Street. Though the shop itself was established in 1908, Selfridges did not have a perfume department until two years later. When the store opened its perfume department it was situated on the ground floor in order to lure the customer in, enticed by the visual spectacle of the sparkling glass bottles and, of course, beautiful and exotic aromas. The positioning of a perfume department near a store entrance to attract customers is still a marketing ploy used by retailers today.

There was a choice of many shops, large and small, from which to buy scents, not forgetting the opportunities offered by mail order and door-to-door selling (in particular from Avon). Perfume companies used all sorts of means to sell their particular brand in the face of stiff competition. Free samples to tempt the buyer were not a twentieth-century phenomenon; remember those little vials known as 'throwaways'. Corday, however, was one of the first perfume houses to trial miniature tubes of its scents attached to bookmarks or illustrated cards. As time went on, the packaging of samples became very sophisticated and by 1952 Corday produced Rue de la Paix, a package in the shape of a Parisian lamppost with three small bottles of perfume inside. The three perfumes were named Fame, Jet and Tzagane, the latter a term for the Romani people.

Aside from samples, free or otherwise, there were other marketing techniques enthusiastically attempted by the fragrance industry. In a nod to cost and practicality, François Coty (1874–1934) chose to make its perfume available in smaller bottles. Fashion designer Jean Patou (1880–1936) offered different scents to match hair colour and invented the perfume bar, where you could mix and match to create your own scent. In the 1950s, Estée Lauder (1908–2004), famous for her scent Youth Dew, which was originally sold as a fragrant bath oil for daily use, came up with the gift-with-purchase idea. Lauder was awarded with the French Legion d'Honneur for her services to the industry. Scented paper fans for advertising perfume were distributed to those hovering at the counter by L. T. Piver, Bourjois and Parfums Rosine to name but a few. Another marketing technique emerged towards the end of the twentieth century when scents associated with celebrities flooded the market. However, while the celebrities themselves were successful the perfumes they promoted did not always do well, as the reader will discover.

Television commercials for perfumes were sometimes controversial and fell foul of the advertising standards regulators; the promotion of Belle d'Opium by Yves Saint Laurent is an example, courting controversy with its hint at drug use. Some perfume advertising was reserved for the American market, such as Catherine Deneuve's campaign for Chanel No. 5. Chanel also made some mini-films to advertise their exclusive wares.

## The Coffret Case: A Special Purchase

It was in the 1900s that perfume houses began to sell samples in elaborate presentation boxes known as coffrets. The coffret or 'small coffer' was modelled on the boxes that often accompanied a bride as part of her dowry in centuries past. However, it was not until the 1950s that these gift items really came into their own. By then, instead of mere samples, the box might contain a full bottle of perfume and a handbag-friendly smaller version as well as an eau de toilette, solid perfume sticks, dusting powder, bath foam, bath cubes, bath salts, soap, hand cream and body lotion all with the same fragrance. An abundance of tissue paper would be used to make an attractive presentation gift and the box beautifully lined and wrapped, perhaps quilted on the inside or even decorated with gemstones, making a coffret case a beautiful and expensive gift.

## What's in a Name?

The name on the label could evoke a memory, offer romance, maybe allude to the sophistication of the wearer and lend a touch of the exotic or the promise of sexual encounter. Think of names like Vol de Nuit, Shalimar, Indiscret, Pompeia and Quelques Fleurs and consider what springs to mind before you have even sampled the fragrance. There were, however, certain curious trends in naming a scent too. For example, there was an oddly prosaic trend for simply giving one's new fragrance a number. Floris 127 and Chanel No. 5 are two famous examples of this fashion. In a further development of this trend, the couture company Balmain's first perfume, created in 1937, took the name Elysees 64-63 from its creator's phone number. Similarly, the cologne 4711, manufactured by the German company Mäurer & Wirtz, was named after the number of the factory in Cologne where it was produced. Made famous by iconic actress Audrey Hepburn, 4711 has survived until the present day without changing its name, its image or its original bottle design. Corday also used her address in naming her collection rue de la Paix. Understandably, the fashion for using addresses and telephone numbers is hardly something anyone would do now when protecting personal data has become so important. French couturier Lucien Lelong (1889–1958) used letters rather than names or numbers to catalogue his perfumes. Presumably the intent was to create an air of mystery that would entice the buyer. At any rate, this was certainly a popular trend in the first half of the twentieth century.

There were, of course, many other ways of choosing a name for your brand or for your new scent. Lancôme opened its exclusive boutique outside Paris in 1935 and took its name from the ruins of the castle Le Château de Lancosme near the region of La Brenne in the centre of France. Armand Petitjean (1884–1969), the founder of the company, had come across the château while on holiday in the region and was intrigued by it and by the roses that grew among its ruins. He used the rose as the logo of the brand. In general, French names for new perfumes continued to be all the rage, promising glamour and a chic style associated with well-dressed and fashionable Frenchwomen.

Perfume houses also maintained the tradition of naming fragrances after particular events or influences of the time too. L. T. Piver's Pompeia of 1907, for example, was named in honour of the ancient Roman town of Pompeii. Guerlain's Djedi, launched in 1926, acknowledged the fascination with Ancient Egypt that was sweeping Europe following the exciting discovery of Tutankhamen's tomb by archaeologist Howard Carter in the same year; the name Djedi is a reference to a magician mentioned in the Westcar Papyrus, a document that dates from somewhere between 1782 BC and 1570 BC. Other companies that had originally established themselves as leaders in selling other luxury goods such as clothing or jewellery, when they entered the perfume market, traded literally on their own name with confidence that it would be enough to sell their new scent. When Tiffany began selling perfume alongside its jewellery in 1987, the company simply called the scent Tiffany, banking on brand recognition.

The names chosen for individual scents became more and more daring and provocative as the twentieth century wore on, reflecting a society that was becoming more liberal and harder to shock or surprise. Some names really did make us sit up and take notice. Dior's Poison is one such case. The hype surrounding this scent did not dissipate on its arrival on the market. Although this might seem a very unusual name for a scent, it actually does fit well with ideas and suspicions about perfume from deeper history.

The bottle in the shape of an apple recalls Snow White, or the biblical story of the forbidden fruit.

## Leather and Cigarettes

The aroma of leather, particularly for men's fragrances, was very popular in the early twentieth century. Raw animal hides were treated with birch tar and boiled to get that woody smell. The Knize Tailoring Company, a Viennese couturier to the court of Kaiser Wilhelm of Germany, produced Knize Ten in 1921, a typically masculine and leathery fragrance. Guerlain's Jicky was a citrusy scent with leathery base notes created in 1889 and is particularly significant. Not only does it define the Jazz Age (it was particularly popular at that time) but to its credit, while countless other perfumes have come and gone, Jicky survives and can be bought today. It is a multifaceted perfume which combines the natural and the synthetic instead of being a one-flower fragrance. The leathery, smoky smell was created by the inclusion of the synthetic coumarin. In Scottish author Compton Mackenzie's controversial novel *Sinister Street* (1913), a dandy named Wilmot smokes a Jicky-scented hookah. By now it had become a more popular fragrance for women as well. Jicky suited the liberated lady, with smoking having become a symbol of female emancipation. The perfume also played into attempts to create a sensual vibe rather than to simply replicate an innocent flower.

By the 1920s, smoking had become quite the fashion with both sexes and it was not unusual to buy cigarettes that had been scented before purchase, perhaps with violet or rose perfume. The arrival of Habanita by Molinard (1921) was something different again. This fragrance was intended not to be applied to a person or their clothing but to a cigarette, which was accomplished by injecting it into the cigarette via a glass rod. A leathery fragrance with a mix of clove, carnation peach and vanilla, Habanita is still on sale today but as a skin perfume.

## Perfume's Criminal Connections

As a valued commodity, perfume was worth stealing (remember Margaret Gainer) either to use yourself or to peddle for a profit. Some 32,000 bottles of eau de cologne were shipped on to the UK in 1908 in one consignment, such was the demand. There are many recorded cases of individuals being convicted of theft of scent in court. In 1907, one William Ludlow, aged twenty, was sentenced at Tower Bridge Police Court in London to two months' hard labour for stealing a box of a dozen bottles of perfume. He was tracked down rather in the tradition of the tales of Marie Antoinette 'by the strong odour of perfume exhaled from his clothing'.

Although we know that whether you like or dislike a certain perfume is a matter of personal preference, the reader might nevertheless be surprised to learn that in 1907 newspapers recalled a brawl in a Berlin tramcar caused by the matter:

> A lady in the car was wearing a scent [that] was so strong that passengers were almost overpowered. The lady's escort showed resentment at the uncomplimentary remarks which were passed and a free fight resulted between the lady's champions and those who objected to the odour of musk. The conductor was obliged to stop the car and call for police assistance whereupon the whole party were taken off to the police station.

## Sinister Scent

Perfume could have sinister connections. Caron's Narcisse Noir, which drove the nuns wild in the 1949 film *Black Narcissus*, and of course Dior's Poison are but two examples. Scent could, in practice, be associated with the dark side just as it had been in the past. The infamous occultist Aleister Crowley (1875–1957) believed scent could not only make him irresistible to women but that the smell motivated men and women to obey his instructions, a means he used in establishing his cult of Thelema. The perfume he wore was called Rutvah, and he referred to it as 'the perfume of immortality'. Rutvah consisted of strong-smelling animal derivatives like civet, musk and ambergris – or perhaps, by this date, their equivalent synthetics. He rubbed this mix into his hair as well as his skin. In an article in the *Penny Illustrated Paper* for November 1910, highlighting Crowley's mystic celebration of what he called the Rites of Eleusis (9 p.m. every Wednesday at Caxton Hall, Westminster), the writer remarks: 'There always has been about his writings and preachings an atmosphere of strange perfume as if he was swaying a censer before the altar of some heathen goddess.' There is little doubt that perfume played a part in enhancing the mysterious and sensual nature of the ceremony, though whether it was the aphrodisiac Crowley thought it was, or how far it influenced his followers, is impossible to know. We can at least say with some certainty that Rutvah did not allow him the immortality he craved.

## Perfume: The Effects of Revolution, War and Conflict

Prior to their downfall in the Russian Revolution of 1917, the Romanov family used perfume as part of their status and mystique. Each of the princesses was alleged to have had their own perfume made especially for them. When the revolution began, perfumers including Ernest Beaux (1881–1961), who had worked for the Romanovs and who would successfully team up with fashion designer Coco Chanel, fled west. Other important Russian émigrés included the Grand Duke Orloff, who would also influence perfume trends in Europe.

Conflict with Germany in the First World War engendered a dilemma: to buy or not to buy. Eau de cologne was originally manufactured in Germany, the enemy country. To resolve this issue, British companies began manufacturing their own eau de cologne, which they claimed was much superior to the German original. Aside from that particular difficulty, shortages inevitably ensued and raw goods such as alcohol were redirected to help with the war effort. The British government clamped down on luxury goods, though they were not too heavy handed when it came to scent. Perfume companies met the government halfway by marketing products with dual purpose. Perfume was even a tool in the war effort in the First World War, as lead acetate hidden in perfume revealed secret ink. The British used this resource to uncover German messages.

America's period of Prohibition from 1920 to 1933, during which the sale of alcohol was forbidden, created a further problem for the perfume industry as there was a shortage of the alcohol essential to the manufacture of modern fragrances. The companies had to argue their case against concerns that they might supply the general public with illegal hooch. To get around any shortages, the perfume company Molinard launched a scent named Concreta in 1925. This was a waxy, solid fragrance produced without alcohol. Long-lasting and available in a range of floral scents (including rose, gardenia and violette), Concreta was advertised as 'the genuine wax of the flowers, used directly as a perfume. Just a touch behind the ear, in the hair, on the eyebrows, on the linings of your coat, is quite enough to be perfumed.' The packaging was made of Bakelite, an easily moulded plastic that was lightweight and synthetic, and came in a variety of shapes including dice, balls, books and flowerpots. These hand-painted containers were fun, appealing and ultimately collectable.

The Second World War brought difficult times for the perfume industry, but although some perfume houses temporarily closed their doors it was not all doom and gloom. Perfume made the wearer feel good. It boosted morale. There was still stock available to purchase. Although there were not many new scents launched during the war, there were some, including the popular Femme de Rochas by Rochas in 1943, which had a warm scent. Powdered perfume that did not need alcohol was also available. Towards the end of the war J. L. Priess marketed Dri-Perfume, which claimed to be a cut above previous dry scents such as the nineteenth-century Frozoclone by Demuth. Just as they did with silk stockings, the American GIs found a way around supply issues and the black market in perfume boomed. Soldiers endeavoured to bring home a bottle of Chanel No. 5 for their loved ones, even if it was a replica and not the real thing.

## Scent and Couture

> That dress fits you wonderfully but one drop of my perfume on its hem and the dress will make you ravishing.
>
> Paul Poiret (1879–1944)

In 1921, fashion designers began to see the possibilities of complementing their quality clothing with their own in-house sophisticated perfumes. Paul Poiret and Coco Chanel (1883–1971), two of the most influential fashion designers of the first half of the twentieth century, took the initial steps with this concept and the idea of a perfume to match one's outfit was born. Poiret, famous for his elaborate fantasy couture gowns, named the perfume arm of his business Perfumes de Rosine after his daughter. At its launch party, dressed in exotic eastern costume, he distributed among his guests bottles of the new scent La Mille et Deuxième Nuit (The Thousand-and-second Night). The scent alluded to the glamorous tale of *A Thousand and One Nights* with all its eastern promise and allure. Other dress designers gained success by labelling their perfumes with the couture name. No doubt associating perfume with high fashion helped maintain the image of scent as luxury item. The high-end market would flourish alongside the new, more affordable brands that arrived in the second half of the twentieth century.

Fashion designer and trendsetter Coco Chanel met the Russian-born Ernest Beaux through her friend Duke Dmitri Pavlovitch (1891–1937), a Russian émigré related to the Czar who was exiled in Paris for his part in the assassination of the monk Rasputin. The duke himself would design the bottle for the ground-breaking scent that Beaux created for Coco Chanel, which was in fact the result of two series of perfumes variously numbered one to five and twenty to twenty-four. Chanel, who believed that 'no elegance is possible without perfume ... it is the unseen, unforgettable, ultimate accessory', chose five as her favourite. Chanel No. 5 boasts more than eighty ingredients and has an androgynous feel about it – a very modern and successful scent synonymous with the ultimate in style.

Others who would join Poiret and Chanel in selling scent to go with their couture outfits included Jacques Fath (1912–1954), Christian Dior (1905–1957), Hubert Givenchy (1927–2018), Paul Balmain (1914–1982) Nina Ricci (1883–1970) and Jean Patou (1880–1936). Christian Dior launched his Miss Dior to accompany his fashion collection, which heralded the feminine and vibrant 'New Look' of 1947; the scent has notes of gardenia, galbanum and bergamot, carnation, iris, jasmine, lily of the valley, rose and narcissus. Miss Dior was named after Christian Dior's sister Catherine. A staunch and active member of the French Resistance during the Second World War, she fell into the hands of the Gestapo and was lucky to survive. Jolie Madame by Balmain (1953) encapsulated in its name the feeling of post-war freedom and was advertised as 'the perfume of adventure for evenings of passion and enchantment' by its creator. Balmain combined this with a clothes collection of the same name. He believed that fragrance was very much part of the whole look. It is still very much the French way to spray or daub perfume onto clothing.

For some dress designers their involvement in the fragrance market outlived their success in the clothing business. This was true in the case of French fashion designer Lucien Lalong (1889–1958), who branched out into fragrance in 1924 after his success in high couture. To begin with his bottles were plain. However, interest grew and with that appeared more lavish containers designed by Lelong himself and based on themes as diverse as architecture and feathers. The mysterious letters that he used as names for his scents and the curiosity as to what was inside the bottles had paid off. In 1948, Lelong abandoned the fashion side of the business but continued to create scent, which he, like so many others in the fashion business, believed was an essential part of feminine style.

## Bottle Design

> The perfume bottles of Paris are irresistible even to the male purchaser.
>
> Walter Kilham (1868–1948)

In the first half of the twentieth century, perfume bottles – and very often the labels on the bottles themselves – were designed by the most well-known artists of the day. French glass designer René Lalique (1860–1945) and the crystal manufacturer Baccarat were particular favourites in the fragrance industry. Both Lalique's bottles and those produced at the Baccarat factory were delicate and expensive in line with their contents, and their designs followed the trends set by the contemporary Art Deco and Art Nouveau movements.

René Lalique got his first commission in 1907 when perfumer, newspaper tycoon and all-round patron of the arts François Coty asked him to design labels for his perfume bottles. Lalique then branched into designing and making the bottles themselves, not only for Coty but other famous perfume houses including Houbigant, Guerlain, L. T. Piver, Roger & Gallet and Worth. In 1924, Dans la Nuit, the first fragrance by Worth, was marketed in a bottle designed by Lalique. Bottles shaped like dresses or the female form stressed the importance of couture designers in their domination of the market.

In 1948, Lalique's son Marc would create one of the most iconic glass bottles of the century for Nina Ricci's scent L'Air du Temps with its distinctive dove-shaped top. Marc's inspiration came from nature and from dance as well as recalling the classical past. These exquisite perfume bottles, designed in the first half of the twentieth century, have held their own to become sought-after collectables in today's art market. Eventually Lalique's descendants were tempted into the perfume industry itself, creating expensive fragrances to match the gorgeous bottles they designed; the feminine floral fragrance Lalique de Lalique was launched in 1992, promising an exquisite scent in an equally exquisite bottle.

## A Night at the Theatre

An outing to the theatre was a popular entertainment and smell continued to feature as part of the performance, whether as a prop or as an element of the plot itself. Perfumes were sometimes named after popular performers. The opera singer Mary Garden (1874–1967) gave her name to a range of fragranced goods that included toilet water, talcum powder, smelling salts and even breath mints. An advertisement for the perfume from 1917 reads, 'Mary Garden Perfume is the original creation of the world's great perfumer Rigaud. Many women are now using the complete set of Mary Garden toilet preparations. There is only one Mary Garden perfume. Every package of Mary Garden toilet requisites bears the name of Rigaud Paris.' The fact that Garden was well known for her rendition of *Salome* and performed the Dance of the Seven Veils herself (this was normally undertaken by a trained dancer) shocked audiences at the time and no doubt endowed the scent bearing her name with erotic connotations. However successful it was as a brand, Rigaud's scent was not without controversy though. It turned out that although the singer had given the perfume house permission to use her name in connection with the perfume, she had not given consent for her portrait to be used in advertisements or for her name to be registered as a trademark. A court case in 1937 would find in Garden's favour.

As far as stage performances go, ballet had a particular association with scent. In 1910 the perfume house Caron produced Isabella, engraved with images of the innovative and highly acclaimed ballet dancer Isadora Duncan (1877–1927). Sergei Diaghilev (1872–1929) and his Ballet Russe toured Europe between 1909 and 1929 to much acclaim, bringing a love of scent and a sense of the oriental with them. The story of ballet

*Le Spectre de la Rose* first performed in 1911 by famous dancers Tamara Karsavina (1885–1978) and Vaslav Nijinsky (1889–1950) centres on the fragrance of a rose. The exotic productions of the Ballet Russes influenced fashion including trends in perfume. Companies launched products with names such as Kismet (Lubin) and the famous Shalimar (Guerlain) that played upon the fascination with orientalism central to a lot of the Ballet Russes' repertoire.

Diaghilev himself loved the scent Mitsouko by Guerlain, referencing the Japanese female name Mitsuko. The perfume is a fine mixture of citrus scents, bergamot, peach, jasmine, may rose, cinnamon, oak moss, vetiver and wood. Diaghilev sprayed the theatre curtains with this scent for the first performance of his ballet *The Rite of Spring* in 1913. Sadly the ballet itself proved too modern for the audience of the time. The perfume, however, was a success.

Antony Tudor (1908–1987) in his ballet *Jardin aux Lilas* (Lilac Garden), first performed in 1936, continued with the perfume theme. In similar style to the impresario Diaghilev, Tudor sprayed the auditorium with lilac perfume for the first performance. By the 1970s others were experimenting with the inclusion of perfume as an element in other forms of art including performance art and installations. Brazilian fabric sculptor Ernesto Neto, for instance, works with stretchy textiles stuffed with spices to create his designs.

## Perfume in the Cinema

Gertrude: Walter, what's that awful smell?
Walter: It's that cologne you gave me for Christmas.
Gertrude: It's lovely, isn't it?

*The Secret Life of Walter Mitty* (1947)

Perfume as a means of promoting a film was not unknown. Vol de Nuit (Night Flight) by Guerlain was launched, or should I say flown, in 1933 to honour Antoine de Saint-Exupéry's novel of that name. A film loosely based on the book, called *Night Flight* but also known as *Dark to Dawn*, arrived on screens in 1933 and spawned a bottle with a propeller stopper. However, on a more subtle level scent meant something whether it was glamour, status, gender, humour, eroticism or even menace.

We can expect perfume to be brought up in scenes of romance or seduction. In *From Russia with Love*, the Russian lady spy sent to seduce James Bond wears Vent Vert by Balmain. It is unclear what Audrey Hepburn wears in the film of *Breakfast at Tiffany's*, but in the novel by Truman Capote on which it is based Hepburn's character Holly Golightly wears 4711. Santa Maria Novella's Melograno, a pomegranate fragrance, features in the Bond movie *Casino Royale*, worn by Bond girl Vesper Lynd (played by actress Eva Green).

There are a few movies where perfume dominates as the subject matter. In Al Pacino's *Scent of a Woman*, for example, the central character is able to recognise a woman by the perfume she wears. The film *Perfume: The Story of a Murderer*, based on the novel by Patrick Suskind, is a story which combines perfume, death and sensuality. In fact, perfume seems to feature more frequently in darker films. This is perhaps an indication of the depth of meaning that can be attributed to it. For example, in *Rebecca* (based on Daphne Du Maurier's novel of the same name), De Winter's new wife is disturbed by the ghostly presence of Rebecca, the previous Mrs De Winter. That presence is suggested by the lingering of Rebecca's signature scent. This is played upon by the menacing Mrs Danvers: 'She looked beautiful in this velvet. Put it against your face. It's soft, isn't it? You can feel it, can't you? The scent is still fresh, isn't it? You could almost imagine she had only just taken it off. I would always know when she had been before me in a room. There would be a little whiff of her scent.' In *The Silence of the Lambs*, serial killer Hannibal Lecter whispers the following words to FBI agent Clarice Starling: 'Sometimes you wear L'Air du Temps ... but not today.' In the movie *Black Narcissus*, a group of nuns relocate to a convent in the Himalayas but are taunted by their past, sensually recalled in Caron's 1911 perfume Narcisse Noir, a scent with exotic and risky connotations.

Like ballet master Sergei Diaghilev, 1930s movie star and sex symbol Jean Harlow favoured Mitsouko by Guerlain, even although that particular scent was intended for brunettes. Although Harlow was a natural brunette, she dyed her hair with caustic chemicals to get her signature platinum-blonde look. In fact, her hair dye would contribute to her early death at the age of twenty-six. Ironically, her perfume, Mitsouko, is sometimes linked with the death of her husband Paul Bern. Shortly after he married Harlow, Bern committed suicide. His body was allegedly discovered drenched in her favourite scent. If true, this paints a tragic yet romantic image of a man in death expressing his undying love for his wife by wearing her perfume.

At the end of the 1950s, filmmakers experimented with Aromarama and Smell o-vision. Reminiscent of the dispensing of saffron around the Coliseum in ancient Rome, Aromarama worked through ventilation systems to create a smell matching what was happening on screen. This was tried for a film called *Behind the Great Wall* in 1958 and proved a dismal failure. Smell-o-vision followed soon after. This time the smells came from vents beneath the cinema seats. It was used for a 1959 film entitled *A Scent of Mystery*. At best failing to work and at worst making members of the audience feel ill, the experiment faltered and failed.

## Scented Oil and the Coronation

The oil used at the coronation of the British kings and queens has a long history. Elizabeth I, who took the throne in 1558, is on record as having detested the smell. Charles I ordered a new, more fragrant version for his coronation in 1626 and it is this seventeenth-century mixture that is closest to the one used at coronations today.

It includes orange blossoms, roses, cinnamon, jasmine, musk, civet and ambergris – quite a mix of the floral and the animal. A large enough batch was made to serve several coronations, but long reigns saw it expire before it could all be used. Queen Victoria's lengthy period of rule necessitated a new batch to be made up for the coronation of Edward VII, the old lot having congealed. While this new batch should have lasted up until the coronation of our present queen, it was destroyed during the war so a further mixture was produced. This time it comprised neroli, jasmine, rose, cinnamon, benzoin, musk, civet and ambergris with a sesame oil base. We have moved some distance from the sacred oil prepared by Moses on God's instructions, but the oil does still require consecration, in this case of the last lot by the Bishop of Gloucester in the chapel of Edward the Confessor.

## Celebrities, Commemoratives and Signature Scent

The actor Rudolph Valentino (1895–1926) caused many women to swoon throughout his short career. He used perfume as part of his role as the eponymous character in *The Sheik* and as a result transformed the image of the American male. Mae West's sensuous figure proved the inspiration for equally erotic bottle shapes and perfume names: Shocking in 1937 by Schiaparelli and Rochas Femme in 1944. The latter was packed in a box lined with black lace reminiscent of a corset that Rochas had made for one of Mae West's film appearances. In 1958, the iconic and glamorous Audrey Hepburn became the first film star to feature as the face of a perfume; in the preceding decades it had been society beauties like Lady Diana Cooper (1892–1986) who had performed this task. Born out of his friendship with Hepburn, however, Hubert de Givenchy (1927–2018) initially created the scent L'interdit (Forbidden) for her. It featured a floral blend of orange blossom, jasmine and tuberose. Imbued with Hepburn's elegance, the perfume was a great success.

Perfumes were still created as they had been in the nineteenth century to celebrate special events. Inspired by Charles

Lindbergh's flight across the Atlantic in 1927, Paul Poiret created Spirit of St Louis. In a bottle draped with the American flag, the perfume was apparently sold 'very much under price'. In 1956, James Henry Creed launched Fleurissimo to mark the fairy-tale wedding of the actress and style icon Grace Kelly to Prince Rainier of Monaco. The special day boasted royalty, romance and Hollywood glamour, and so did the scent with its mixture of bergamot, tuberose, violet, iris, Bulgarian rose and ambergris. Creed had designed the fragrance to complement the bride's bouquet. Schiaparelli, meanwhile, sent a bottle of Le Roi Soleil (The Sun King) to Wallis Simpson, Duchess of Windsor, when she was exiled in Paris. 'It is really the most beautiful bottle ever made,' wrote the duchess. 'It has displaced the duke's photograph on the coiffeuse.' Given Wallis's reputation in the media at the time, and the hurt caused by her husband abdicating the throne to marry her, this endorsement may have been a bit of a double-edged sword. Nonetheless, she was an independent and modern woman and from that point of view her recommendation would have been of value.

When the general populace got to know that a certain perfume was preferred by a celebrity, such an association could benefit a brand. Apparently Elvis Presley wore Brut by Brut and Frank Sinatra was partial to Yardley's English Lavender Soap, while heavy metal icon Ozzy Osbourne used No. 88 by Czech and Speake. John F. Kennedy favoured Eight and Bob by Albert Fouquet, Princess Diana wore Bluebell by Penhaligon's and of course Marilyn Monroe famously wore Chanel No. 5 and nothing else – not in bed, anyway.

While some celebrities clearly associated themselves with certain perfumes, in the closing years of the twentieth century many promoted scents under their own name. Elizabeth Taylor's White Diamonds (1991) for women and Antonio by Antonio Banderas (1997) for men certainly made a profit. However, success as a performer did not guarantee the same in the perfume market. Elvis's Love Me Tender, produced in 1970, might be good memorabilia but it was not a hit as a perfume. The general view is that so-called celebrity perfumes are rather tacky and do not have the provenance of fragrances marketed by the well-established houses.

## The New Twentieth-century Perfume Houses

Many companies experimented with scent in the twentieth century. Some survived, and some didn't. The picture is more blurred than it had been in the past as many of the companies that began to make perfumes also manufactured other items, particularly high fashion clothing and makeup. However, most of the companies discussed in this book were, and in most cases still are, almost exclusively perfume sellers.

First there is Coty, founded in 1904 by Francois Coty, who became known as the 'Napoleon of Perfume'. Coty set a trend for spicy florals at mid-market prices. He exploited synthetics and supported the emancipation of women. He was good at marketing his products and understood the importance of naming and presenting his perfumes to attract attention. He paid attention to the packaging, establishing a profitable partnership with glassmaker René Lalique, whose bottle designs were more than worthy of their contents at the time and are very much sought after as collectable items in their own right today. Perfume was not Coty's only business, but it made him a lot of money. He also owned newspapers, including *Le Figaro*.

Next we come to Volnay, founded in 1919 by the adventurous Germaine and René Duval. René had worked for Coty while his wife Germaine, when not away on some adventure (she was the first woman to fly over the Andes, albeit as a passenger) was a model for Lanvin, the fashion house founded by Jeanne Lanvin in 1889. The Duvals travelled the world in search of fine ingredients. The first perfume they produced was called Yapana (1922), named after an aromatic plant from Latin America that was believed to have healing properties. All Volnay fragrances have a powdery rose, vanilla and clove base which is part of their unique identity.

Corday, founded in 1924 by Blanche Arvoy, was named after Charlotte Corday (1768–1793), who assassinated the French revolutionary Marat and was subsequently executed. The company was one of the first to promote its wares through samples. When composer Harry Revel (1905–1958) met a woman in a hotel lobby he was so taken with the Corday perfume she wore that he set six Corday fragrances to music: Toujours Moi, Tzigane, Possession, L'Ardent Nuit, Jet and Fame. The company was sold to the makeup giant Max Factor in 1961.

Fragonard, founded by Eugene Fuchs in 1926, was named after French artist Jean-Honoré Fragonard (1732–1806). The name is also a subtle tribute to the perfume hub that is Grasse – the painter Fragonard hailed from that town.

Of course, there will always be new entrepreneurs daring to try their hand in the lucrative perfume business. Among the most recent are the Cotswold Perfumery, which specialises in bespoke perfumes, Diptyque, the brainchild of a painter, an interior architect and a theatre set designer, and finally Tiziana Terenzi, an Italian firm that stresses the importance of perfume in relation to emotion and memory.

## Landmark Scents: The Taglines

'When you have nothing to wear' – Je Reviens by Worth.

'When crystals sparkle like diamonds ... when cider tastes like champagne ... you are under the spell of...' – Evening in Paris by Bourjois.

'Things don't happen the way they used to but they still happen' – Tabu by Dana.

'Gives you the time of your life' – Charlie by Revlon.

'Are you her type?' – L'heure Bleue by Guerlain.

'The most expensive perfume in the world' – Joy by Patou.

'Even in the dark he'll know it's you' – Intimate by Revlon.

'Who wears Muse shares the secrets of the goddesses' – Muse by Coty

# THE TWENTY-FIRST CENTURY
## What Next?

The appeal of perfume is that it is at once ephemeral and
empowering. It creates a shimmering invisible armor that lingers in
a room long after its wearer has gone and infuses our imagination
with a subtle power, hinting at a hidden identity.

Mary Gaitskill (1954–)

Today scent is everywhere. We liberally use room fragrances and
perfumed soaps in our homes and offices. Paris and New York
subways employ scent to counteract the smell of crowded bodies
waiting for their trains. Car air fresheners are commonplace.
The wide range of perfumes at an equally wide range of
prices makes a dab of perfume accessible to almost anyone.
The ubiquitous nature of fragrances, however, comes with a
certain loss of exclusivity of taste in perfume today. The market
is driven not by quality but by celebrity culture, advertising and
consumerism. This has drawn criticism. In *The Times*, columnist
Hannah Betts described perfumes in 2003 as 'insipidly unisex eau
de celeb, too many thinly veiled takes on laundry detergent'.

However, the appeal of scent is long-lasting and the expensive
end of the perfume market still spells the ultimate in luxury. No. 1

by Clive Christian (previously the Crown Perfumery Company) is better known as simply 'the most expensive perfume in the world'. Launched in 2006, No. 1 for women has Indian jasmine and Tahitian vanilla, tonka bean seeds, sandalwood, cedarwood and musk. The equivalent for men combines lily, sandalwood, pink grapefruit, heliotrope, mandarin and lime. In addition, there is a limited edition of the scent known as No .1 Imperial Majesty, of which only ten bottles were ever produced. Price is available on request, and the bottle itself is made from crystal and gold. A royal connection also lends prestige to Christian's; their latest scent is 1872, a mix of mandarin and neroli, named for the year in which Queen Victoria gave the Crown Perfumery Company permission to use the crown on its bottles in perpetuity. The perfume itself recalls the romance of Victoria and Albert's love match in an era when marriages among the elite were not made for love.

Thankfully, the romantic image of perfume, if not its aristocratic associations, does stretch across the range of goods available. A cheap or expensive bottle of perfume is still a suitable gift for loved ones on a birthday, at Christmas or on Valentine's Day.

We are happy today to accept what people of the past, particularly in the ancient and classical periods, always knew: that fragrance has health benefits, including stress reduction, better sleep, improved mood and better performance at work. However, we no longer rely on scent to prevent or treat disease. On the contrary, in the twenty-first century we are more likely to worry about perfume inflaming allergies.

Perfume remains relevant in religious contexts, albeit restricted to certain belief systems. Economically, too, it remains a major feature. Clearly there is still money to be made, and persuading the customer to buy through attractive packaging, special offers and free samples is the name of the game. It has also continued to be cited in intrigue, too. In the case of the Salisbury poisonings of 2018, the nerve agent Novichok was found in a bottle of

Premier Jour by Nina Ricci. It was because the packaging was recognisable and connoted expense that the unintended victim picked it up.

Many of the ingredients in perfume, putting aside the more recently invented synthetics, have remained unchanged over centuries; even a cursory look along the perfume and cosmetic counters in a twenty-first-century department store or specialist perfume shop will make that abundantly clear. Many of the smells appreciated by people as far back as the Bronze Age are still very much in favour today: rose, jasmine, violet, orange blossom. However, the emphasis has moved away from worship and medicine to glamour and self-expression.

Many of the new perfumes on the market today trade on names that recall ideas long associated with fragrance alongside modern trends, from traditional floral scents like Dolce & Gabanna's Dolce Rose Eau De Toilette or Daisy by Marc Jacobs to perfumes expressing modern independence and individuality such as My Way by Armani. Other scents from the past have stood the test of time and remain popular, like Chanel No. 5 or Miss Dior. In truth, scent has never lost its relevance or its mystique. Proust said it best: 'Perfume is that last and best reserve of the past, the one which, when all our tears have run dry, can make us cry again.'

# GLOSSARY OF INGREDIENTS

**A**

| | |
|---|---|
| Absinthe | A herb, also known as wormwood. See Artemisia. |
| Acacia | Gum Arabic. This is a natural resin. |
| Agarwood | The source of this scent is a fungal infection that grows on a tall evergreen tree called the Aquilaria. Agarwood is also known as aloeswood or agallochum, though it is more often referred to today as Oud. |
| Agrimony | A herb whose yellow flowers and leaves are used in perfumery. |
| Aldehyde | Aldehydes are organic compounds found naturally in many plants. These can be replicated artificially. |
| Alkanet | A red dye extracted from the root of a small, herb-like tree native to the Mediterranean and Asia Minor, used in scent to make the product more appealing. Also known as bugloss or anchusa. |

| | |
|---|---|
| All-heal | Any of several plants believed to have healing properties of which valerian is one. |
| Almond | A species of small tree. Almond oil is extracted from the fruits. |
| Aloeswood | See Agarwood. |
| Amber | In the classical world this refers to a fossil resin. However, in modern perfumes it refers to a sweet mix of scents. |
| Ambergris | A secretion from the intestines of the sperm whale produced as a reaction to the texture of their diet of crayfish. The name means 'grey amber'. A wax-like substance that smells very unpleasant (faecal in fact) when fresh but as it matures becomes sweet and woody. |
| Ambrette | Oil distilled from the seeds of the musk mallow. Musk-like smell. |
| Ambrosia | Oil from a herb known as Mexican wormwood. Geranium-like smell. |
| Ambroxan | A synthetic substitute for ambergris. |
| Anchusa | See Alkanet. |
| Angelica | A scented herb. The name means 'Herb of Angels'. Aromatic oil is extracted from the seeds, leaves, stems and roots of the plant. |
| Anise | A Mediterranean herb of the parsley family with liquorice-flavoured seeds. Oil of anise is distilled from the seeds. |
| Apple | Popular in early Arabic scents. |
| Apple blossom | Essence from various species of apple tree is popular, particularly those with cherry-pink or white petals. |

| | |
|---|---|
| Apricot | Oil extracted from both the flesh and kernel of the apricot is used in perfumery. |
| Artemisia | Herbaceous plant, also known as wormwood or mugwort. The name means sacred to the goddess Artemis. |
| Asafoetida | A bitter gum resin is extracted from the root of this tall herbaceous plant. |
| Ash | The leaves and bark of the ash tree are popular. |
| Aspalathus | A shrubby herb with aromatic leaves, aspalathus is also the source of rooibos tea. |
| Attar | Anglicized Arabic term for perfume, traditionally meaning the mixture of floral or other fragrant material mixed with an oil base. This is a term applied to rose essential oil in particular. Also known as Otto. |

**B**

| | |
|---|---|
| Balanos oil | Fragrant oil extracted from a thorny tree known as the Egyptian plum tree. |
| Balm of Gilead | A resin from the balsam poplar tree. The name refers to the ancient region of Gilead in Palestine. |
| Balm of Judea | Botanical identity not known. The balm is thought to have had a lemony smell. |
| Balm of Peru | An aromatic resin from the trunk of the *Myroxylon balsamum* tree. |
| Balsam | A general term for gum resin from various trees and shrubs. A thick but not solid substance used as a base for medications and perfumes. |

| | |
|---|---|
| Barberry | The red berries of the plant *Berberis vulgaris*. |
| Basil | A garden herb. The name in ancient Greek means kingly. |
| Bay leaf | Oil is distilled from the leaves of the bay tree. |
| Bdellium | An aromatic gum from trees of the genus *Commiphora*. Similar to myrrh. |
| Benjamin | See Benzoin. |
| Ben oil | See Moringa oil. |
| Benzoin | A gum generated by the damaged bark of trees of the genus storax. Also known as Benjamin. |
| Bergamot | The rind of the fruit from a small, spiny tree produces a citrus-scented oil. The plant also has highly scented white flowers. The fruit resembles a small green orange but is not edible. |
| Betony | A herb belonging to the mint family. |
| Bishopswort | See Betony. |
| Bitumen | A tarry substance with a strong odour. |
| Blue lotus | *Nymphaea caerulae* or blue waterlily. |
| Borage | A herb with blue flowers and hairy stem. The leaves are cucumber-scented. |
| Boxwood | An ornamental tree of which the dried bark is used. The wood is hard and light yellow. |
| Brimstone | Largely used as a fumigant in the pre-modern world, this is a fine powder of sulphur. |
| Broom | A dense shrub with fragrant yellow flowers. |

## C

| | |
|---|---|
| Calamint | A bushy herb. A camphorous essential oil is extracted from the leaves. |
| Calamus | A water plant whose rhizomes give off scent. Name means 'reed' in Ancient Greek. In ancient times 'calamus' may have referred to lemongrass or sedge. Also known as sweet flag. |
| Camomile | The name means 'earth apple', referring to the apple scent of the flowers when dried. |
| Camphor | The granular, crystalline substance produced by the wood of the camphor tree. A very aromatic gum. |
| Caraway | A herb with aromatic seeds similar to fennel. |
| Cardamom | A perennial shrub native to India and Sri Lanka. Sometimes referred to as 'the grains of paradise'. The seeds give the scent. |
| Carnation | Clove pink. This is sometimes referred to as the gillyflower. |
| Cashmeran | A synthetic substitute used in perfumes. This is a complex odour intended to suggest the softness of cashmere wool. |
| Cassia | The Cassia tree originated in China. The bark is used in the same way as cinnamon; the two are often confused in Greek and Roman texts. Cassia is of lesser quality. |
| Castoreum | An oil from the glands in the groin of the beaver. This was used as a perfume fixative. |
| Cedarwood | A fragrant hard wood from the cedar tree, a tall conifer. |

| | |
|---|---|
| Celery | Oil is harvested from crushed seeds of the wild celery plant. |
| Centaury | All of this herbaceous plant is useful. The genus includes knapweed and cornflower. |
| Cinnamon | Comes from two trees native to central Asia. The yellowish-brown bark is dried and used in a range of perfumed goods to this day. |
| Citronella | A grass with lemon-scented leaves from which aromatic oil is extracted. |
| Civet | A paste-like substance extracted from the gland under the civet cat's tail. This has a strong faecal fragrance on its own. |
| Clary sage | A herb. Clary is derived from the Latin *clarus*, meaning clear. |
| Clover | The honey-like smell of clover blossoms is now replicated synthetically. |
| Cloves | An East Indian evergreen tree. The unopened flower buds are used whole or ground into a powder. |
| Cockle | A shellfish. Ground shell may have been used in a powdered scent. |
| Coconut | Oil is extracted from the fruit of the coconut tree. |
| Comfrey | A hairy-leaved plant. The leaf and root have been used in perfumery. |
| Coriander | A herb with aromatic seeds native to the Mediterranean. |
| Cornflower | See Centaury. |
| Costmary | A herb native to Asia which has aromatic leaves. The plant, a member of the daisy family was regarded as sacred to the Virgin Mary; hence its name. |

| | |
|---|---|
| Costus | A minty perennial. The scent comes from the root. |
| Coumarin | A synthetic. The chemical is found naturally in sweet clover and in tonka beans, the fruit of a flowering tree of the pea family. |
| Cowslip | A type of primrose. The yellow flowers are prized for their apricot scent. |
| Crocus | See Saffron. |
| Cumin | A small herb with aromatic seeds. |
| Cyperus | Sedge root related to papyrus. Also known as galingale or nut grass. |
| Cypress | Oil from the leaves and twigs of the cypress tree. |

**D**

| | |
|---|---|
| Daffodil | See Narcissus. |
| Daisy | Both the flowers and leaves of this common flower are used. |
| Dill | An aromatic garden herb. |
| Dock | Also called monk's rhubarb, this is a broad-leaved weed. |
| Dragant | An aromatic gum. |

**E**

| | |
|---|---|
| Elecampane | A member of the sunflower family. The roots produce an oil. |
| Eucalyptus | Aromatic oil is extracted from the leaves of the Eucalyptus tree. |
| Euganol | A synthetic substitute for clove oil. |

**F**

| | |
|---|---|
| Fennel | The aromatic seeds of this herb were used in perfume and medicines. |

| | |
|---|---|
| Fenugreek | Native to south-eastern Europe and western Asia, the seeds of this herb are aromatic. |
| Flax | The source of linseed oil. |
| Forget-me-not | A plant with small blue flowers that are lightly fragrant in the morning and at night. |
| Frangipani | A tropical flowering tree. Named after a perfume created in the Renaissance period because the said tree has a similar smell – a strange case of the perfume preceding the flower. |
| Frankincense | Gum resin from olibanum trees of the genus *Boswellia*. The tree is native to Arabia, Somalia, Ethiopia and India. |

## G

| | |
|---|---|
| Galbanum | A bitter aromatic gum resin, semi-solid or solid, collected from the stems of the giant fennel. Native to Persia. |
| Galingale | An Indonesian plant with a rhizome similar to ginger but rose-like in its perfume. |
| Gallnut | This is also known as the oak apple, a deposit formed by insects on the leaves of oak trees. |
| Gardenia | The flowers of this shiny-leaved exotic plant produce a scent. |
| Geranium | Oil is extracted from the flowering plant of that name. |
| Germander | An aromatic herb that is a member of the mint family. |
| Ginger | A reed-like Asian plant with an aromatic root. |
| Ginger grass | Similar to lemongrass. |

| | |
|---|---|
| Gladiolus | A popular garden plant with tall spikes. The smaller flowering variety has a scent. |
| Gorse | A shrub with yellow flowers that have a vanilla-like fragrance. |
| Grapefruit | The peel of the fruit is used in potpourri and quality scents. |
| Gum arabic | See Acacia. |

## H

| | |
|---|---|
| Hartshorn | The ground horns, hooves or bones of the red deer. |
| Hartwort | A herb. Member of the carrot family. |
| Heliotrope | A family of flowers with a vanilla fragrance. |
| Hemp agrimony | A tall plant with pink and purple flowers. |
| Henbane | A poisonous plant. |
| Henna | A small shrub with fragrant flowers. |
| Honeysuckle | A shrub. An essential oil is extracted from the flowers. |
| Hyacinth | A powerful scent is extracted from the flowers of this popular perennial plant, which is grown indoors and outdoors. |
| Hyssop | A woody evergreen herb with aromatic leaves as well as fragrant flowers and stems. The name means 'holy herb' in ancient Greek. |

## I, J, K

| | |
|---|---|
| Ionone | A synthetic that replicates the scent of violets. |
| Iris | This is a water plant named after Iris, the Roman goddess of the rainbow. A powder is made from the plant roots. |

| | |
|---|---|
| Jasmine | Also known as jessamine, the plant has fragrant white flowers and aromatic leaves. Jasmine has a low yield and cannot be synthetically produced. |
| Jessamine | See Jasmine. |
| Jonquil | See Narcissus. |
| Juniper | The cones of the juniper tree are aromatic. A fragrant oil is also extracted from juniper berries. |
| Knapweed | See Centaury. |

**L**

| | |
|---|---|
| Labdanum | This is a gum sourced from the underside of the leaves of the rock rose. |
| Laurel | A volatile oil is extracted from this small tree native to the Mediterranean. The aromatic berries are used, as is the sweet-scented wood. |
| Lavender | The fragrance comes from oil extracted from the fresh flowering tops of the lavender plant and also from the stalks. |
| Lemon balm | A herb. It attracts bees with its scent and so has another name, Melissa, derived from the Ancient Greek for 'honeybee'. |
| Lily | Madonna lily or Annunciation lily yields scent from its flowers. |
| Lily of the Valley | The scent comes from the small, bell-shaped flowers of this plant. |
| Lime | Fragrant oil is extracted from the fruit rind of the lime tree. |
| Linseed | Oil from the flax seed. |
| Lupin | A tall garden plant with flowers that come in many colours. |
| Lye | Caustic soda. A waxy white solid. |

## M

| | |
|---|---|
| Mace | See nutmeg. |
| Mallow | The flowers and the leaf of this plant have been used in perfumery. |
| Marigold | Also called Calendula. The flowers give a small amount of fragrant oil. This can also be used to colour a product. |
| Marjoram | A bushy annual herb. An essential oil can be obtained from the flowers and leaves. Together with oregano, the herb was known as Origanum by the Romans. |
| Mastic | A gum extracted from the bark of the lentisk tree. |
| Maudeline | Sweet-scented yarrow. The flowers and leaves of this common wildflower have been used for their fragrance. |
| May blossom | The flower-bearing hawthorn. |
| Meadowsweet | A wildflower. The scent comes from the flower buds, which have an almond-like fragrance. |
| Melilot | See sweet clover. |
| Melissa | See Lemon Balm. |
| Mimosa | The sweet-scented yellow blossom of the mimosa tree. |
| Mint | Perennial spearmint or peppermint. There are a number of other varieties including horsemint, garden mint and pennyroyal. |
| Moringa oil | The seeds of the moringa tree produce a high yield of oil; also known as ben oil. |
| Moss | Lichen with a woody, earthy smell. |
| Mugwort | See Artemisia. |
| Musk | The glandular secretion of the male musk deer. |

| | |
|---|---|
| Myrrh | A bitter gum resin. From a small tree *Commiphora myrrha*, native to Arabia and East Africa. |
| Myrtle | The leaves, twigs and flowers of this shrublike tree all exude fragrance. |
| Myrobalanum | See Moringa oil. |

**N**

| | |
|---|---|
| Nabk | A thorny, shrub like tree. |
| Narcissus | The white flowers from this tree are used in perfumery. The narcissus family includes the daffodil. |
| Nard | A flowering plant of the honeysuckle family. The rhizomes or underground stems of this plant are crushed and distilled to produce thick oil. There are Syrian, Indian and Celtic varieties. |
| Nasturtium | The leaves and stems of this trailing plant are used for their scent. |
| Neroli | The essential oil from the flowers of the bitter orange tree. |
| Nutmeg | The dried kernel of the seed from this tree is used. |
| Nut grass | See Calamus. |

**O**

| | |
|---|---|
| Oakmoss | A lichen found growing on oak trees and popular in perfumery. |
| Olibanum | See Frankincense. |
| Omphacium | Oil from unripe olives or dates. |
| Onycha | The name means 'sweet hoof'. The plant appears in the Bible as an ingredient in holy incense but is unidentified to date. |
| Opobalsamum | See Balm of Judaea. |

| | |
|---|---|
| Opoponax | Gum resin from the Bdellium trees, sometimes referred to as myrrh. Lavender-like fragrance. Juice is extracted from the base of the stem. |
| Orange blossom | The fragrant flower of the orange tree. See also Neroli. |
| Oregano | A herb. |
| Orris | A powder made from the roots of the iris, a decorative perennial. Violet-like scent. |
| Oud | See Agarwood. |

**P, Q**

| | |
|---|---|
| Patchouli | An essential oil with a musty, earthy aroma from an East Indian bushy herb. |
| Pennyroyal | A perennial herb of the mint family. |
| Persimmon | An extinct plant much valued in the classical period. |
| Petitgrain | The oil from the leaves, twigs and unripe fruit of the bitter orange tree. |
| Pine | The oil from the twigs and needles of the pine tree. |
| Poppy | This flower has a heavy odour when fresh. |
| Pot ash | Plant ashes or wood ashes soaked in a pot. |
| Quince | The fruit and the blossom yield a fragrance. |

**R**

| | |
|---|---|
| Resin | The hardened secretions of plants. A translucent, brittle substance. |
| Rhodium | See Rosewood. |
| Rockrose | See Labdanum. |
| Rose | The most popular plant in perfume history. Scent extracted from the petals. |

|  | Rosewater is the steam distillation of roses or rose petals infused in water. |
| Rosemary | Aromatic shrub with fragrance from the flowers. |
| Rosewood | A tropical tree with a reddish bark and yellow or pink flowers. |
| Rue | A strong-scented evergreen herb native to the Mediterranean. |

## S

| Safflower | Oil from seeds and dye from flowers of a thistle-like plant. |
| Saffron | Dried stigma of the crocus. |
| Sage | A shrubby evergreen herb. Oil is extracted from the flowering tops of the plants and from the dried leaves. |
| Saltpetre | Potassium nitrate. Once a fumigant, this white powder is now used as fertilizer. |
| Sandalwood | The fragrance taken from the roots and bark of a small evergreen tree called the Sandal tree. The tree needs to be at least thirty years old before it yields any oil. |
| Sassafras | The dried wood bark or root of the sassafras, a deciduous North American tree. |
| Satinwood | A sweet wood. |
| Savory | Herb with an aromatic mint fragrance. The twigs and leaves are the source. |
| Sedge | See Calamus and Sweet Flag. |
| Sesame oil | Extracted from the seeds of the flowering sesame plant. |
| Seselis | See Hartwort. |
| Southernwood | A small shrub related to wormwood. The flower tops have a lemony scent. |

| | |
|---|---|
| Spikenard | See Nard. |
| St John's wort | Essential oil is extracted from the flowers of this plant. |
| Storax or styrax | Gum resin from a small deciduous tree native to southern Europe and the Middle East. |
| Sweet cane | A grass. |
| Sweet clover | A fragrance comes from the white and yellow flowers of this plant. |
| Sweet flag | See Calamus. |
| Sweet reed | A marsh plant. |
| Sycamore | Fig fragrance. |

**T**

| | |
|---|---|
| Tacamahaca | The North American and East Asian poplar tree. A balsam is extracted from its buds. |
| Tansy | A herb of the aster family with edible flowers. |
| Terebinth | An aromatic resin extracted from the Pistacia tree. Sometimes called turpentine. |
| Thyme | A perennial herb. |
| Thyron | A reed or rush. |
| Tonquin | The flowering tree of the pea family that produces tonka beans. |
| Tragacanth | A resin is extracted from this thorny shrub. |
| Tuberose | A bulb that produces white, lily-like flowers from which scent is extracted. |
| Turmeric | The powdered root of the turmeric plant. |
| Turpentine | Any of various resins from coniferous trees. |

## V

| | |
|---|---|
| Valerian | A herb. The dried roots yield oil. See All-heal. |
| Vanilla | An essence from the seed pod of the vanilla orchid. Requires extensive processing to produce a scent. |
| Vanillin | A synthetic substitute for vanilla. |
| Vervain or verbena | The scent from leaves and flowers of a perennial plant with pale lilac flowers. |
| Vetiver | An oil is distilled from the fibrous root of this grass. |
| Violet | A small perennial plant. Scent is derived from the flowers. |
| Viper's bugloss | A bristly plant with bright blue flowers. |

## W

| | |
|---|---|
| Wallflower | A herb with scented flowers. Also known as the gillyflower. |
| Watercress | A leafy vegetable. |
| Water lily | A water plant. |
| White horehound | A flowering plant of the mint family. |
| Willow bark | The bark from several varieties of willow tree. |
| Woodruff | A new-mown hay fragrance comes from the dried leaves of this plant belonging to the madder family. |
| Whortleberry | A fruit-bearing plant. |

## X, Y

| | |
|---|---|
| Xylobalsamum | See Balm of Gilead. |
| Yarrow | See Maudeline. |
| Ylang-ylang | An aromatic Asian tree. The fragrant, greenish-yellow flowers yield an oil used in perfume. |

# SELECT BIBLIOGRAPHY

I have made use of a considerable number of primary sources in the writing of this book. Information about these sources is contained within the text itself.

Aftel, Mandy, *Essence and Alchemy: A Book of Perfume* (New York: North Point Press, 2002)

Dayagi-Mendels, Michal, *Perfumes and Cosmetics in the Ancient World* (Jersualem: The Israel Museum, 1989)

Dugan, Holly, *The Ephemeral History of Perfume: Scent and Sense in Early Modern England* (Baltimore: John Hopkins Press, 2011)

Ellis, Aytoun, *The Essence of Beauty* (London: Secker and Warburg, 1960)

Fornaciai, Valentina, *Toilet Perfumes and Make-up at the Medici Court: Pharmaceutical Recipe Books Florentine Collection and Medici Milieu Uncovered* (Livorno: Sillabe 2007)

Groom, Nigel, *The Perfume Handbook* (London: Chapman and Hall, 1992)

Lyttelton, Celia, *The Scent Trail: An Olfactory Odyssey* (London: Bantam Press, 2002)

Manniche Lisa, *Sacred Luxuries: Fragrance Aromatherapy and Cosmetics in Ancient Egypt* (Ithaca, New York: Cornell University Press, 1999)

Maxwell, Catherine, *Scents and Sensibility: Perfume in Victorian Culture* (Oxford: Oxford University Press, 2017)

Morris, Edwin T., *Scents of Time Perfume from Ancient Egypt to the 21st Century* (Boston: Metropolitan Museum of Art, 1999)

Muchembled, Robert and Pickard, Susan (trans.), *Smells: A Cultural History of Odours in Early Modern Times* (Cambridge: Polity, 2020)

Ostrom, Lizzie, *Perfume: A Century of Scents* (London: Penguin Random House, 2015)

Perry, Charles (trans.), *Scents and Flavors: a Syrian Cookbook* (New York: New York University Press, 2020)

Reinarz, Jonathan, *Past Scents: Historical Perspectives on Smell* (Champaign: University of Illinois Press, 2014)

Rimmel, Eugene, *The Book of Perfume* (1865)

Stewart, Susan, *Cosmetics and Perfumes in the Roman World* (Stroud: Tempus, 2007)

Turin, Luca and Sanchez, Tania, *Perfumes: An A-Z Guide* (London: Profile, 2009)

Verrilll, A. Hyatt, *Perfumes and Spices* (Redditch: Read Books Ltd, 2013)

Wilson, C. Anne, *The Country House Kitchen Garden 1600–1950* (Stroud: Sutton, 2003)

# ACKNOWLEDGEMENTS

My grateful thanks go to Alicia Shultz of LBCC Historical Apothecary (http://www.etsy.com/ie/shop/LitttleBits) in particular for what I consider to be one of the most interesting images in the book. Thank you too to Hillary, Curator of the Make-up museum (http://www.makeupmuseum.org) for all her help and support. I acknowledge that I found the details about General Wade's Balsam in Vivienne Gabrielle Hatfield's PhD thesis 'Domestic Medicine in Eighteenth Century Scotland' (awarded in 1980), which quoted from the private papers of Lady Catherine Stewart. I do not claim to have had sight of the original source in this case.

Thank you to Amberley Publishing for agreeing to produce a second book with me and in particular to Shaun Barrington and Alex Bennett for being there on the other end of emails despite the ups and downs of the Covid epidemic. I hope this volume is a worthy companion to *Painted Faces: A Colourful History of Cosmetics*.

Finally, as ever, I would like to thank all of my family for their patience and enthusiasm.

# INDEX